PREPARING
FOR PANDEMICS

Lessons from the
Global Financial Crisis and COVID-19

PREPARING
FOR PANDEMICS

Lessons from the
Global Financial Crisis and COVID-19

David Longworth • Frank Milne

Queen's University, Canada

World Scientific

NEW JERSEY · LONDON · SINGAPORE · BEIJING · SHANGHAI · HONG KONG · TAIPEI · CHENNAI · TOKYO

Published by

World Scientific Publishing Co. Pte. Ltd.

5 Toh Tuck Link, Singapore 596224

USA office: 27 Warren Street, Suite 401-402, Hackensack, NJ 07601

UK office: 57 Shelton Street, Covent Garden, London WC2H 9HE

Library of Congress Control Number: 2022019350

British Library Cataloguing-in-Publication Data
A catalogue record for this book is available from the British Library.

PREPARING FOR PANDEMICS
Lessons from the Global Financial Crisis and COVID-19

ISBN 978-981-125-592-2 (hardcover)
ISBN 978-981-125-593-9 (ebook for institutions)
ISBN 978-981-125-594-6 (ebook for individuals)

For any available supplementary material, please visit
https://www.worldscientific.com/worldscibooks/10.1142/12825#t=suppl

Desk Editor: Lai Ann

Typeset by Stallion Press
Email: enquiries@stallionpress.com

TO OUR WIVES AND GRANDCHILDREN
Hoping that the world will be better prepared the next time

Anne and Margaret

Alan, Craig, Justin, Gemma, and Mabel

This book is a winner on two fronts: it is badly needed and it is very interesting. No country was even close to being adequately prepared for Covid-19, though some in the developed world, including Canada, thought they were, because of lessons learned from SARS in 2003. But there is vastly more to pandemic preparation than storing away some PPE, and those preparations extend far beyond just the health care system. What they are, and how they can be conceived, modelled, and tested is what this book is about. It should be read and followed. We need to be able to do better next time.

John Scott Cowan, PhD
Retired Medical Research Scientist and Principal Emeritus,
The Royal Military College of Canada

With Covid-19 showing hopeful signs of subsiding and the prospect of a return to the "new normal", authors Milne and Longworth call for much-needed preparedness for the inevitable next pandemic. It's a fascinating analysis. By comparing the current situation with the Global Financial Crisis of 2007–2009, they draw attention to the vital matter of avoiding the dreadful mistakes made in the handling of today's crisis and applying the lessons learned. This they propose through a logical process of data-collection, post-mortem analysis, war-gaming, simulation, and application. It's a huge challenge, calling for massive international cooperation in numerous areas touching on more than simply the medical aspects. The very nature of global politics and diplomacy will be put to the test. Will it be an opportunity to show that democracy outplays oligarchy in applying the lessons of Covid-19 and its variants? Will ethics dilemmas (think anti-vax) be resolved the next time around?

For a better understanding of how the impact of future pandemics can be minimized, one would do well to read, study and apply the authors' superb analysis and support their conclusions.

General (Ret'd) **Paul Manson**, O.C., C.M.M., C.D.
Chief of the Defence Staff 1986–89

Longworth/Milne's book extracts lessons from plans to deal with crises, notably that of global finance in 2007/9, and the current viral pandemic. If learned and applied, they could diminish applicability of the adage that even best-laid plans "gang aft agley". The authors' principal recommendations are for the establishment of powerful standing authorities to do penetrating "post mortems" on existing pandemic and other plans and in planning for future crises of all kinds, to conduct regular stress tests and war-games, well-established tools of the financial and military worlds. The predictive results should deal with the breadth of the impact of a future crisis on every jurisdiction, health, economic, financial, social, cultural, overall well-being and, above all, be designed to counter complacency, the nemesis of crisis preparedness.

Duncan G. Sinclair
Professor emeritus, Queen's University

The idea behind this book is tremendous: that policy makers should learn from disasters and crises in other fields, not only their own. That imperative is addressed with expertise, and judicious intelligence. This is an important book which policymakers, commentators, and scholars should take seriously.

Paul Tucker
Harvard Kennedy School
Former central banker

Covid-19 has been plaguing the world now for more than two years. Enough time has now passed to start reviewing mankind's performance in managing it. David Longworth and Frank Milne have taken an interesting multi-disciplinary approach to such a review by comparing the Covid-19 Global Pandemic to the Global Financial Crisis. This enables them to draw out a richer set of lessons from the similar shortcomings that emerged from the two crises than one might find by simply reviewing the pandemic from a public health management perspective. I commend their book and approach to all both from the standpoint of gaining a better understanding of how this pandemic could have been better managed, and as a template as to how such multi-disciplinary reviews can be conducted in the future.

Mark Zelmer
C.D. Howe Institute
Former prudential regulator

Contents

About the Authors

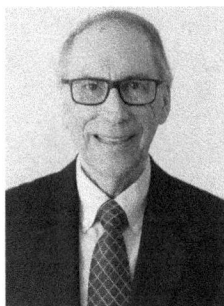

David Longworth was a Deputy Governor of the Bank of Canada in the financial system area from 2003–2010, at the end of a 36-year career there. As a Deputy Governor, he served as a member of the Governing Council of the Bank. During the Global Financial Crisis, he was the Bank's representative on the Committee on the Global Financial System and the Markets Committee, which meet at the Bank for International Settlements.

He has been a Term Adjunct Professor in the Department of Economics at Queen's University since 2011, where he also served as Associate Director of the Graduate Diploma Program in Risk Policy and Regulation from 2014–2018. He has taught courses there in comparative credit cycles, financial regulation, and advanced topics in risk management and regulation. From 2010–2020, he was also Adjunct Research Professor at Carleton University, frequently teaching a course on central banking.

David Longworth graduated with a PhD in Economics from MIT in 1979. He has published in leading journals, including the *Journal of Finance*. His major research interest is financial regulation, especially dealing with systemic risk through macroprudential policy. He is a Research Fellow of the CD Howe Institute.

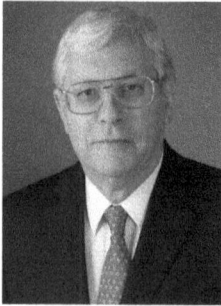

Frank Milne graduated with a PhD from the Australian National University in 1975. He has held positions at the University of Rochester, the Australian National University, and the Australian Graduate School of Management. He joined the Queen's Department of Economics in 1991. In July 2000 he was appointed to the BMO Chair in Economics and Finance, and more recently he was the Director of the Risk Policy and Regulation graduate program in the Queen's University Department of Economics.

He has published many papers in leading economics and finance journals. For many years he has acted as an advisor and consultant for various branches of the Australian and Canadian governments. In 2008–2009 he was a Special Advisor at the Bank of Canada during the financial crisis.

Acknowledgments

For a book that is multidisciplinary, we were very fortunate to be able to draw on experts in many fields, including public health, financial regulation, governance, financial risk management, credit and bankruptcy resolution, catastrophe insurance, stress tests, and wargames. In particular, our book benefitted immensely from e-mail discussions with several individuals. John Cowan raised a number of points related to the COVID-19 pandemic and read an early draft of Chapter 2. Drawing on their experience during the global financial crisis and the subsequent improvements in financial regulation, Mark Zelmer and Larry Schembri made a great number of useful comments on a draft of Chapter 3, including ones that informed improvements we made to other chapters. Paul Tucker's comments on a draft of Chapter 4 greatly improved our discussion of governance and the roles of independent agencies. John Crean (in his joint work with Frank Milne) helped us understand the significant role that catastrophe insurance and its interaction with bank credit systems can play in reducing the economic and financial costs of future pandemics. Kevin Dowd read a draft of Chapter 5 and made comments on stress tests. The book's analysis is much stronger because of the contributions of all these individuals. All weaknesses, errors, and omissions that remain are our own.

We would also like to thank our editor, Lai Ann, for her patient guidance, and the other staff at World Scientific Publishing who were involved in the editing and publishing of this book. The book reads and looks much better for it.

Our wives, Anne and Margaret, supported us greatly during this two-year writing project, for which we are very grateful.

Chapter 1

Introduction: COVID-19 and the Authorities

By the end of 2021, the COVID-19 pandemic had led to the third largest loss of life due to a pandemic since 1900, exceeded only by the "Spanish influenza" of 1919–1920 and HIV-AIDS. It was also associated with the largest decline in economic output since the Great Depression of the 1930s and very large government deficits. Avoiding such extreme outcomes in the future will require careful analysis of the successes and failures of policy actions.

Twelve and a half years before the start of the pandemic, another world event was attracting attention — the beginning of what became known as the Global Financial Crisis (GFC). It became evident that financial regulators and governments in advanced economies had not done enough to avoid, or at least dampen, such an event.

In the first few months of the COVID-19 pandemic, it became increasingly evident that public health authorities and governments — at both national and state/provincial levels — were not well prepared. This lack of preparation included dealing with factors which affected the spread of the disease itself, as well as broader health issues such as mental health and delayed surgeries. However, it also encompassed government policy issues related to providing income and loan supports, as well as implementing various types of lockdown restrictions and school closures.

There are many parallels between the lack of preparation for COVID-19 and the unpreparedness of financial regulators prior to the GFC. These include the following: failing to have sufficient stocks of equipment, supplies, space, and staff (or, in the financial crisis, of equity capital and liquidity); a clear understanding of how much of such resources can be borrowed, and from which organization and under what circumstances, or obtained from abroad; data collected and shared in a consistent manner across health units and sub-national governments (banks or countries); clear early warning systems, including sharing what is found; plans for dealing with contagion from abroad; a clear understanding of operational risks that themselves require preparatory steps to deal with; an understanding that individuals are diverse and that this heterogeneity needs to be take into account in modeling; and an understanding that planners need to take into account behavior outside the highly regulated part of the health (or financial) system, such as in long-term care homes (and shadow banks).

Since there are so many parallels between the two crises, there are serious lessons to be learned from the changes made after the GFC. Those lessons plus the governance, legitimacy, and transparency of planning for future pandemics is the focus of this book.

Those lessons should be applicable to most economies, but our focus is on advanced democratic countries. Our examples throughout are largely drawn from the United States, the United Kingdom, Canada, and Australia — the last two with which we are most familiar. As three of these four nations are federations, they also struggled with split responsibilities for managing the pandemic between the federal and state (provincial) levels.

It is important to note that there was one significant difference between the preparations for the COVID-19 crisis and the financial crisis: Much of what was needed to be done in terms of the health side of pandemic preparation was well known and documented in reports on previous epidemics (SARS, H1N1, MERS, and Ebola) and planning documents. However, in a number of countries, much of the planning had never led to concrete actions before COVID-19.[1] This points to a major governance failure. It also raises the question as to whether independent agencies

---

[1] See, for example, Global Preparedness Monitoring Board (2019).

should be created to carry out postmortems, draw up and implement plans, and provide ongoing monitoring of their implementation.

In 2022, it will be important for governments and public health authorities to carry out broad-based postmortem reports on the pandemic to provide lessons for the updates of pandemic plans. Those reports should also deal with governance and transparency issues. The discussion of governance will need to deal with the legitimacy of the structure being proposed[2]: What is the role of legislating (the legislature), drawing up and testing plans (perhaps by independent agencies), monitoring (by auditors general and the like, as well as legislative committees), and implementing fully funded plans (by the executive and public health authorities)? Although the details will differ across countries because of the various natures of their constitutions and governing structures, there are principles regarding legitimacy, accountability, and transparency that should be observed in democracies. The details are important, because governments (and the public) tend to over-discount the future ("hyperbolic discounting"), and therefore steps to create credible commitments to actually carry out pandemic preparation plans will improve societal welfare. Put another way, resilience has been undervalued in the past but deserves much more attention as a societal value. Broad-based postmortems also need to take into account sustainability (including government finances), as well as fairness in health services and who pays the economic costs.[3]

In addition to the broad-based postmortems, it will be necessary for hospitals, public health authorities, educational institutions, mental health institutions, and associations of health professionals to conduct more detailed reviews on very specialized topics.

Some postmortems on important topics have already appeared. For example, the Canadian auditor general issued several chapters of her 2021 report on government responses to the pandemic.[4] Among other topics, she recommended that the Public Health Agency of Canada improve its information technology infrastructure, better promote timely risk assessments, and improve systems for nationwide mandatory quarantines. At the

---

[2] See Tucker (2018) for a detailed discussion of the key issues.
[3] Carney (2021).
[4] Auditor General of Canada (2021).

international level, there has been an independent panel report on some of the shortcomings of the World Health Organization and the global response.[5]

This is a good start, but much of it has been limited to a subset of health system responses: It does not address the implications of other government policies, such as those related to lockdowns, which have impacted important aspects of society and the economy. Broader postmortems require careful analysis of government policy responses, their successes and failures. The failures require serious attention, whether they were related to the lack of preparation going into the pandemic or policy failures during the pandemic. It is critical that lessons learned are incorporated into recommendations for dealing with future pandemics. These recommendations need to be based on evaluations of alternative policies for future pandemics — including under which circumstances they would be appropriate. Those evaluations need to include broad considerations, including lost schooling and intergenerational equity. Recommendations need to be incorporated into formal plans, which then need to be implemented.

Plans should also incorporate what has been learned from the experience of other countries, including, but not limited to, during the COVID-19 pandemic. There appear to be some clear lessons from South Korea and Taiwan during the pandemic, as well as from Japan's experience with an annual day for disaster prevention, which involves millions of citizens in drills as well as preparation by many senior government officials. Regular training programs for key personnel, as well as annual reminders to the public that all of us need to be prepared, should be considered.

The plans also need to be regularly tested. Stress tests and exercises (sometimes known as wargames) have been found to be extremely useful ways of testing plans in many different areas. These include the military, the financial sector, corporate strategy, and public health. They are used to discover areas where preparedness is currently insufficient. A stress test examines the effect of a large negative event on health, social, and/or economic systems to test its resilience. This technique has been used extensively by private banks and bank regulators to test the solvency of banks

---

[5] Independent Panel for Pandemic Preparedness and Response (2021).

and banking systems. Indeed, another parallel between the lack of preparation prior to the pandemic and the experience of regulators before the GFC was that the stress tests were not as expansive and stressful as they should have been. Subsequently, such tests in the financial sector were greatly improved.

In the pandemic preparation area, a stress test could consist of having an external party create a plausible scenario, but one that is fundamentally different from what has happened in the recent past. This could include an assumed new disease, spread in a particular way, affecting certain age groups, with a particular degree of transmissibility. The stress test should include the social, economic, and other consequences of government action (e.g., the consequences of a lockdown over a specific period of time). The entire stress test should be revealed at once and officials should take sufficient time to work through all the implications in some detail, consulting across agencies and sections within agencies to ensure that the response is consistent. This can be important in breaking down silos, which are a major problem in large organizations dealing with new challenges.[6] After the response to the stress test is submitted, weaknesses in current plans should be noted and recommendations to improve them should be made to the government and the appropriate legislative committee and then made public. Follow-up on those recommendations is essential.

An extension of the stress test idea is an exercise. This technique extends the idea of a stress test to a real-time simulation of a crisis, such as a pandemic, with the participation of very senior officials (those who would be making decisions or recommendations during an actual pandemic) from government health and treasury/finance departments, as well as from the public health agency. This exercise should explore the accuracy and timeliness of information systems and the effectiveness of decision-making procedures. This is important, because in the COVID-19 pandemic, information and other systems in many jurisdictions have been found wanting. Generally, it should be carried out over a short period of time such as a day or a weekend. New information about the pandemic scenario should be revealed by the organizers at various points of time during the exercise period to simulate essential learning.

---

[6] See Tett (2015).

As in the case of stress tests, such exercises were carried out both in the financial system prior to the financial crisis and in the health system prior to the pandemic. However, in both cases, they were insufficiently expansive. The pandemic exercises that have been run have tended to be limited to particular aspects of the health system. They have not incorporated the wider implications for broader public health issues and government actions related to the details of lockdowns, as well as fiscal and monetary policies. Furthermore, there has been a very disturbing lack of implementation of recommendations from previous limited health exercises, which points again to weaknesses in governance.

In the next four chapters of the book, we thoroughly examine each of the issues described above. The poor preparation for the pandemic is discussed in Chapter 2. The parallels between this poor preparation and the behavior of financial regulators prior to the GFC are the subject of Chapter 3. Chapter 4 deals with the construction of postmortems for the COVID-19 pandemic as well as constructing plans for the preparation for future pandemics. Importantly, it discusses the role of governance, legitimacy, and transparency in helping to ensure that the plans are actually put into place. Chapter 5 follows with how the processes of stress tests and exercises can help to improve plans over time. Chapter 6 concludes.

References

Auditor General of Canada (2021). *2021 Reports 6 to 8, 10 and 11, and 12 to 15.* https://www.oag-bvg.gc.ca/internet/english/parl_lp_e_933.html.

Carney, M. (2021). *Value(s): Building a Better World for All.* Penguin Random House Canada.

Global Preparedness Monitoring Board (2019). "A World at Risk," Annual Report 2019, September.

Independent Panel for Pandemic Preparedness and Response (2021). "COVID-19: Make it the Last Pandemic," May.

Tett, G. (2015). *The Silo Effect: The Peril of Expertise and the Promise of Breaking Down Barriers.* Simon & Schuster, New York City.

Tucker, P. (2018). *Unelected Power: The Quest for Legitimacy in Central Banking and the Regulatory State.* Princeton University Press, New Jersey.

Chapter 2

Poor Pandemic Readiness

1. Introduction

Much was revealed in the first half of 2020 regarding the relative unpreparedness of Public Health Authorities and their governments in many countries, even in those where extensive reports had been written in response to earlier pandemics or epidemics.[1]

In this chapter, we focus on weaknesses in the planning and preparation of the Public Health Authorities — and associated weaknesses in government planning and preparations — given what has been revealed by the COVID-19 pandemic. Weaknesses in planning and preparation have likely significantly increased the health, economic, and social costs of the pandemic.

There is pervasive uncertainty in an epidemic or pandemic associated with a new disease, regarding important details about the transmission of the disease and who is at greatest risk of dying; elements of that uncertainty can last for several months. Another fundamental uncertainty is how

---

[1] See the 2020 Annual Report of the Global Preparedness Monitoring Board (GPMB), https://apps.who.int/gpmb/assets/pdf/200913_GPMB_2020_Annual_Report_press_release.pdf. "In its new report, the GPMB provides a harsh assessment of the global COVID-19 response, calling it 'a collective failure to take pandemic prevention, preparedness, and response seriously and prioritize it accordingly.' In many countries, leaders have struggled to take early decisive action based on science, evidence and best practice. This lack of accountability by leaders has led to a profound and deepening deficit in trust that is hampering response efforts."

the public will react to any policy that has never before been put into place. It is impossible to define optimal policies *ex-ante*. However, uncertainty can be magnified if known existing vulnerabilities (such as inadequate hospital space and inappropriate conditions in long-term care facilities) have not been dealt with or if appropriate planning is not done in advance. Key areas need to be covered in such a planning exercise, including the following:

- Allocations of responsibility;
- How key actions would be carried out;
- Requirements for equipment, personnel, and space in worst-case scenarios;
- Expectations of the public at large and private sector organizations; and
- Communication procedures with the public at large and private sector organizations, as well as among governments, public health authorities, and medical personnel.

In undertaking planning, authorities need to be cognizant of the fact that the response of the public to the perceived seriousness of disease (not only the probability of death but also the probability of severe illness) will lead to changes in behavior even in the absence of any policy implementation by public health authorities or government. These changes could include reducing travel (local public transport, national, and international), avoiding crowded situations (including non-essential shopping), pulling children out of school, and refusing to work in situations that are felt to be unsafe.

Section 2 of this chapter deals with shortcomings in the public health preparation for pandemics. The early months of the COVID-19 pandemic showed the **absence** of the following:

- A plan for sufficient availability of personal protective equipment, ventilators, other equipment, workers, and hospital space during a pandemic.
- Clarity of expectations for non-health-sector employers regarding personal protective equipment.

- Clarity in federations or countries with regional health authorities of the role of the national government in providing additional personal protective equipment and ventilators.
- Clarity of policy tools regarding closure of borders to people.
- Examination of operational risks in important elements of the health care sector.
- Clear strategy for testing for a disease and contact tracing in the case of communicable diseases.
- Clear standards for rapid detailed data collection and report dissemination regarding (i) disease and (ii) total deaths in the economy.
- *Ex-ante* consideration that possible policies to contain the disease may have on (i) mental health and (ii) delaying surgeries for serious health conditions.
- *Ex-ante* consideration of how messages should best be communicated to the public, for example, to limit unwanted effects on mental health and the amount of physical exercise.
- *Ex-ante* consideration of how to deal with workplaces, especially in key industries, where physical distancing is difficult given current work practices (especially where a "production line" is involved).
- Comprehensive advanced warning systems.

These shortcomings all became evident within a few months of the confirmation by the World Health Organization (WHO) that we were indeed in a public health emergency of international concern on 30 January 2020. We illustrate many of these shortcomings with experience from around the world, with particular attention given to the United States, the United Kingdom, Canada, and Australia.

In Section 3 of the chapter, we deal with shortcomings in government preparation for pandemics. The first categories of shortcomings are those related to weak oversight and inadequate funding of health departments and public health authorities. Just as important, there appears to have been a lack of appreciation by most governments of how they would be pulled into making key decisions when a pandemic broke out. There was often little *ex-ante* appreciation (1) that health, social, and economic factors are interdependent, and (2) that there were economic and fiscal preparations that governments needed to make to deal with a variety of major shocks, especially pandemics. Examples of the first are joint consideration by public authorities on limiting social interaction (outdoors and inside) and limiting economic interaction (workplace and marketplace). Examples of the second are consideration of how to get income and loans to a huge number of people (and then how to phase out that support), and more explicit planning to understand economic linkages and to list those industries that are absolutely essential. Governments also needed to be better prepared to pay particular attention to the plight of low-income and disadvantaged racial groups.

Even after the first few months of the official pandemic, further shortcomings in procedures became evident. We explore some of these issues in Section 4. These included failing to learn from the first wave of the pandemic and from experiences in other countries, in preparation for subsequent waves. In addition, some countries seemed ill prepared to consider appropriate strategies for ordering vaccines. Finally, there was not a coherent world strategy to vaccinate those residing in poor countries, which would both reduce the chances of more major mutations and increase the demand for and supply of world vaccine output.

Appropriate preparation by public health and governments involves having appropriate models in place — both epidemiological models and models that capture the interactions between public health, the economy, and health and government policy. Models are always simplifications of the real world. However, severe oversimplifications can lead to poor policy and poor forecasts, as we discuss in Section 5. We are particularly concerned that prior to the pandemic there were few models that (i) emphasized important heterogeneities across the population and locales, and their implications for policy, and (ii) could be used to examine overall economic and social costs — as opposed to just the direct impact of a pandemic on morbidity and mortality — associated with policy responses.

Section 6 concludes the chapter and introduces the idea of parallels with another major shock.

2. Shortcomings in Public Health Preparation for Pandemics

In principle, pandemics can occur in many types of infectious diseases (communicable diseases). They can be contagious diseases spread by contact with infected individuals or their bodily fluids or discharges, by contact with objects or surfaces that have been contaminated by such fluids or discharges, or by ingesting contaminated water or food. They can also be the type of infectious diseases that arise from direct or indirect contact with insects (e.g., mosquitoes or fleas) or animals (mice). In the advanced world, pandemics have occurred in the form of contagious diseases spread by contact with infected individuals or their bodily fluids or discharges (directly or indirectly through contaminated objects or surfaces). Most pandemics in advanced economies since the beginning of the 1900s have been from contagious viruses, particularly influenza viruses and coronaviruses. Pandemics from these two types of viruses will be the focus of much of our paper, but much of our writing applies to pandemics more broadly.

We outline eleven major shortcomings in preparation for a pandemic in many advanced economies.

2.1 *Plans for equipment, buildings, and labor not made or not implemented*

Dealing with risks of any kind typically requires a plan (not just a report) that is adopted by the relevant authority or board. A key element of this plan is specifying how the additional services required ("surge capacity") when a pandemic occurs will be produced from equipment, buildings, and labor. This would often involve establishing a stockpile of required equipment and, often, excess accommodation for patients. This should include plans specifying under what conditions additional personnel will need to be hired and existing personnel redeployed.

When the COVID-19 pandemic hit, in a large number of jurisdictions, many health workers did not have sufficient personal protective equipment (PPE) such as N95 masks, shields, and gowns, thus endangering their health. This shortage was recognized by the World Health Organization (WHO) on March 3, 2020.[2] This shortage was largely because countries like Canada[3] and the United Kingdom[4] had let their stockpiles run down, while others, like Australia,[5] had not taken pandemic scenarios into account in establishing the targets for stockpiles.

Moreover, there was a perceived lack of ventilators to treat the very ill, including in Australia, Canada, the United Kingdom, and the United States.[6] There was also a lack of testing kits, in part because of a shortage of key inputs into those kits such as swabs and reagents (testing chemicals).[7] (Furthermore, there was no plan as to how domestic production of needed equipment could be ramped up immediately.)

In this pandemic, a number of jurisdictions, including many Canadian provinces, started with hospitals very close to full capacity. (To make

---

[2] World Health Organization, "Shortage of Personal Protective Equipment Endangering Health Workers Worldwide," 3 March 2020.

[3] See Rachel Gilmore and Mahima Singh, "Feds Continue to Seek Masks, Other PPE After Admitting Stockpile 'Likely' Not Enough," *CTV News*, 2 April 2020. https://www.ctvnews.ca/health/coronavirus/feds-continue-to-seek-masks-other-ppe-after-admitting-stockpile-likely-not-enough-1.4880269; and Evan Dyer, "The Great PPE Panic: How the Pandemic Caught Canada with its Stockpiles Down," *CBC News*, 11 July 2020.

[4] Harry Davies, David Pegg, and Felicity Lawrence, "Revealed: Value of UK Pandemic Stockpile Fell by 40% in Six Years," *The Guardian,* 12 April, 2020; and Haroon Siddique, "What is the Situation with Personal Protective Equipment in the UK?" *The Guardian,* 14 April 2020.

[5] Matt Woodley, "Government 'Did Not Consider' Pandemic Risks on PPE Stockpiles: ANAO," *newsGP,* 11 December 2020.

[6] ABC News, "Coronavirus Pushes Government to Commission 2,000 New Ventilators for Australian ICUs," 8 April 2020; Kerri Breen, "Coronavirus Pandemic Puts Canada's Supply of Ventilators in the Spotlight," *Global News*, March 17 (updated March 20), 2020. https://globalnews.ca/news/6682780/coronavirus-pandemic-ventilators-canada/; Adrian O'Dowd, "COVID-19: Government was too Slow to Respond to Ventilator Shortages, Say MPs," *The BMJ*, 25 November 2020; and "Critical Supply Shortages — The Need for Ventilators and Personal Protective Equipment during the COVID-19 Pandemic," *The New England Journal of Medicine*, 30 April 2020 (published 25 March 2020 on the journal's website).

[7] See Andrew Russell, "Coronavirus: How Rapid Testing Kits could Lead to More Targeted Screenings," *Global News*, April 6 (updated April 13), 2020. https://globalnews.ca/news/6785112/coronavirus-rapid-COVID-19-test-kits-canada/.

hospital beds available for what might be needed for COVID-19 patients, all elective surgeries were to be cancelled.) Other jurisdictions, such as the United Kingdom and United States, went into the pandemic in much better shape, with capacity problems expected to be relatively minor and perhaps localized.[8] Some new hospital rooms were constructed, in places such as Wuhan, China;[9] Hamilton, Ontario;[10] and London, England, and other spaces were converted to provide testing facilities. There was an attempt to expand the capacity in New York in cooperation with the U.S. military, but the initial stages of the expansion were botched.[11]

Also, in many Canadian provinces, there was already a shortage of personal support workers, especially in long-term care facilities (nursing homes). In part, this was because of poor working conditions, low pay, no benefits, and the hiring of many part-time workers who had two or three jobs in different long-term facilities (Dijkema and Wolfert, 2019; Working Group on Long-Term Care, 2020). When some personal support workers caught COVID-19, there were not enough other personal support workers to replace them. This led to hospitals having to lend personnel and Quebec and Ontario requiring support from the Canadian Armed Forces.[12]

As new information becomes available (e.g., from epidemics elsewhere, and the availability of new types of equipment), plans need to be revised to take this information into account.

---

[8] Ruth McCabe, Nora Schmit, Paul Christen *et al.*, "Adapting Hospital Capacity to Meet Changing Demands during the COVID-19 Pandemic," *BMC Medicine,* 16 October 2020; and Doug Badger and Norbert Michel, "Coronavirus: Policymakers Should Augment Hospital Capacity where Needed, Not Mandate Permanent Excess Capacity," Backgrounder No. 3487, The Heritage Foundation, 16 April 2020.

[9] See BBC News, "Coronavirus: The Hospital Built in a Matter of Days," February 2, 2020. https://www.bbc.com/news/in-pictures-51280586.

[10] See Dan Taekema, "How to Build a Hospital Wing for a Pandemic in just 14 Days," *CBC News*, April 2. https://www.cbc.ca/news/canada/hamilton/covid-joseph-brant-blt-construction-pandemic-unit-1.5518090.

[11] See The Washington Post. https://www.washingtonpost.com/national/javits-center-comfort-new-york-covid-patients/2020/04/10/edeb002e-7a82-11ea-b6ff-597f170df8f8_story.html.

[12] See Emma McIntosh, "Ottawa to Send Military to Help in Ontario Nursing Homes Hit by COVID-19," *Canada's National Observer*, April 23, 2020. https://www.nationalobserver.com/2020/04/23/news/ottawa-send-military-help-ontario-nursing-homes-hit-covid-19.

2.2 Unclear public health authority expectations for the non-healthcare sector

The assumptions that authorities make about the behavior and preparedness of the public need to be communicated clearly to the public.

In many (especially non-Asian) countries, members of the public were unaware of the potential advantages of non-medical masks and so did not generally own any. Some large employers in Canada did own significant numbers of non-medical masks and PPE, for example, Bell Canada (2020), but this was the exception rather than the rule. Even long-term care homes did not have sufficient PPE for their employees. It is not clear whether employers in the food, agricultural, and fishing industries had ever been asked to think about acquiring PPE for their employees prior to COVID-19. Even in August and October 2020, surveys by Statistics Canada showed that roughly 40% of Canadian businesses were still concerned about shortages of personal protective equipment.[13]

2.3 Absence of clarity of stockpiling roles of various levels of government

Clarity of roles in a federation or in a country where there are regional authorities needs to be established.

Although constitutions lay down the responsibilities for health, even where the responsibility for health is a state/provincial one, the federal government often takes on certain roles, even if it is a coordinating one. From an insurance point of view, it is cheaper for some of an equipment stockpile to be held at the federal level so that the equipment can be made available to the states or provinces needing it. However, there needs to be clarity *ex-ante* of the appropriate sizes of stockpiles so that one level of government is not assuming that the other will be doing nearly all of the provision of equipment. Such *ex-ante* clarity is also important when there is only one level of government, but regional health authorities exist and

---

[13] Statistics Canada, "Navigating the Second Wave: Trends in Businesses' Needs for Personal Protective Equipment Since August," StatCan COVID-19: Data to Insights for a Better Canada, 14 December 2020.

have been given some role in targeting and holding stockpiles of needed equipment. The purpose of stockpiles also needs to be made clear. A Canadian government official argued that the federal government's stockpile was not designed for a pandemic[14] and senior White House advisor Jared Kushner claimed at one point that the U.S. federal stockpile was not meant for states.[15]

Cooperation between national and provincial or regional governments in procurement of necessary equipment would also be helpful, especially if agreed to in advance. In Australia, the Auditor General argued that the federal Department of Health should collaborate with states in documenting priorities for procurement.[16] In the United Kingdom, Scottish and Welsh cabinet ministers were concerned in April 2020 that England was being prioritized by private suppliers, perhaps with instructions from the national government.[17]

2.4 *Insufficient advance discussion of policy tools regarding borders*

No matter what shock we are talking about, a large percentage comes from abroad. Therefore, border policies are an important issue.

Pandemics by their very definition start in one country and spread abroad. Pandemics of contagious diseases, especially influenza and coronavirus diseases, are almost always going to be spread by international travellers. Thus, countries need to think *ex-ante* about prohibition of travel versus quarantine. In the latter case, they need to consider how quarantine is to be implemented (including reports, location, and enforcement). In principle, travel restrictions are to be governed by International Health

---

[14] See Ryan Tumilty, "Government Officials Say National Stockpile Not Designed for Pandemic: 'We Do Not Focus on PPE'" *National Post*, May 15, 2020. https://nationalpost.com/news/government-officials-say-national-stockpile-not-designed-for-pandemic-we-do-not-focus-on-ppe.

[15] Nicole Lyn Pesce, "Jared Kushner Slammed for Saying the Federal Medical Supply Stockpile isn't Meant for States," *MarketWatch*, 3 April 2020.

[16] Matt Woodley, *op. cit.*

[17] Libby Brooks and Steven Morris, "Scotland and Wales Concerned Over Reports England is Prioritised for Coronavirus PPE," *The Guardian*, 14 April 2020.

Regulations (2005) and associated recommendations by WHO. Many countries did not follow the WHO's recommendations from 29 February 2020,[18] but it has been argued that one should not assume that they violated international law.[19]

It is unclear if, prior to the pandemic, many countries had plans or options regarding borders, especially on what should guide the decisions to prohibit certain types of travel and the type of quarantine that should be implemented. In the COVID-19 pandemic, a number of "island nations" such as New Zealand and Australia moved fairly quickly to close borders, while other countries (e.g., the United Kingdom) were much slower in closing borders. There are various policy options available, and some may be more successful than others. For example, some have pointed to Hong Kong's model, involving testing and quarantine, as being preferable to a mode such as Canada's.[20] Because of the potentially important economic and diplomatic effects of border closures or restrictions, national governments need to be prepared to take decisions in a timely fashion.

Restricting travel across state or provincial boundaries or across regions within geographically large provinces or states should also be considered *ex-ante*. Canadian Atlantic provinces and Canadian territories either closed their borders or required a two-week quarantine.[21] The provinces of Quebec[22] and British Columbia, the Australian states, and the

---

[18] World Health Organization, "Updated WHO Recommendations for International Traffic in Relation to COVID-19 Outbreak," 29 February 2020.

[19] Barbara von Tigerstrom and Kumanan Wilson. (2020). "COVID-19 Travel Restrictions and the *International Health Regulations (2005)*," Commentary, *BMJ Global Health,* 5(5); and Caroline Foster, "Justified Border Closures do not violate the International Health Regulations 2005," *EJIL: Talk!* 11 June 2020.

[20] See The Globe and Mail, "Hong Kong Stopped a Pandemic at the Border. The Trudeau Government has to Do the Same," May 14, 2020 for May 15 Newspaper. https://www.theglobeandmail.com/opinion/editorials/article-hong-kong-stopped-a-pandemic-at-the-border-the-trudeau-government-has/.

[21] See CBC News, "As Provincial Governments Ease Lockdowns, Many Travel Restrictions Remain," May 11, 2020. https://www.cbc.ca/news/canada/provinces-travel-restrictions-border-checkpoints-1.5561074.

[22] CBC News, "Quebec Restricting Travel to 'Vulnerable Regions' as it Works to Contain COVID-19," March 28, 2020. https://www.cbc.ca/news/canada/montreal/covid19-march28-1.5513555.

country of Italy are three other examples, among many, which restricted travel across regions in their jurisdictions.

2.5 *Insufficient consideration of operational risks*

Any firm or government needs to consider operational risks. There are some key operational risks presented by contagious diseases when health care workers work in two or more locations and/or come into contact with many people outside of work. In Canada and other countries, there are many nurses and personal support workers, as well as some doctors, who work in more than one hospital or long-term care facility. This has helped the spread of COVID-19. Such work arrangements do not appear to have been considered *ex-ante* in Canada. The Office of the Public Health Officer (2020) in British Columbia banned personal support workers from working in more than one facility early in the pandemic. It took other Canadian provinces, such as Ontario, longer.[23] There also should be *ex-ante* advice for health care workers as to their contact with people outside their facility, considering the possibility of contagion in both directions. The massive, deadly outbreaks in long-term care facilities in many countries have raised serious questions about the readiness and rate of adoption of best practices in such facilities.[24]

Another operational risk is not having enough laboratory capacity to process tests for a disease. This was a problem in the Canadian province of Ontario,[25] the United Kingdom,[26] and the United States.[27]

---

[23] DeClerq, Katherine, "Ontario Restricts Long-Term Care Home Workers to One Facility Amid COVID-19 Pandemic," *CTV News*, April 14, 2020. https://toronto.ctvnews.ca/ontario-restricts-long-term-care-home-workers-to-one-facility-amid-COVID-19-pandemic-1.4895852.

[24] Madalina-Gabriela Barbu, Christina Beiu, Liliana Gabriela Popa *et al.*, "The Impact of COVID-19 Pandemic on Long-Term Care Facilities Worldwide: An Overview on International Issues," *BioMed Research International*, Hindawi, 11 November 2020.

[25] The Globe and Mail, April 16, 2020.

[26] Jacqui Wise, "COVID-19: What's Going Wrong with Testing in the UK?" Feature Briefing, *The BMJ*, 21 September 2020.

[27] Willem Marx, "COVID-19 Testing Capacity Strained by Surge in Demand," *NBC News*, 5 December 2020.

2.6 *Insufficient planning for testing and contact tracing*

All organizations should want to know the size of the problem, how fast it is growing, and how the problem is spreading (both the big picture and the details).

For contagious diseases, health authorities need to know the total number of cases, how fast cases are growing, and how the disease is being transmitted (both person-to-person and at particular locations such as conferences, workplaces, and long-term care facilities). This requires both lots of testing and tracing the contacts of those who test positive.

Lack of test kits can be a problem in doing adequate numbers of tests. Initially, this can be because of the time it takes to develop an adequate test and make sufficient test kits. But later, it can be because of poor preparation in having the materials and manufacturing capacity necessary to make the test kits and having enough laboratory capacity to process the tests. This appears to have been the case in both Canada and the United States — at least in some provinces and states. The amount of testing has varied greatly across provinces,[28] states (Johns Hopkins Coronavirus Resource Center, 2020), and countries (Our World in Data, 2020).

Testing should ideally be given to all persons experiencing symptoms, health care workers who are in contact with those who have been infected, and samples of people who reside or work in risky facilities (e.g., long-term care facilities, retirement homes, grocery stores, and meat processing plants.) As well, there should be a daily random sampling from the general population so that the true spread in the population can be known, as well as the proportion of those infected who are showing no symptoms.[29] In Canada[30] and many other countries, this standard has not been consistently

---

[28] CBC News "Regional Testing" May 28, 2020, updated daily, https://newsinteractives. cbc.ca/coronavirustracker/.

[29] Eric Hoskins, "Is COVID-19 Less Lethal than We Thought?", Opinion, *The Globe and Mail*, published May 14 (online) and May 15 (print), 2020. https://www.theglobeandmail. com/opinion/article-could-covid-19-be-less-dangerous-than-we-thought/.

[30] Michael Wolfson, "During the Pandemic, why has Canada's Data Collection Lagged so Far Behind?", Opinion, *The Globe and Mail*, published April 13, 2020, updated April 14, 2020. https://www.theglobeandmail.com/opinion/article-during-the-pandemic-why-has-canadas-data-collection-lagged-so-far/.

met throughout the crisis. In principle, widespread random testing can provide data useful for building better models of the spread of a pandemic.

When there are few cases and they have mostly come from abroad, contact tracing can be easier because there are lots of public health resources available (and for new cases, the infected often know if they've been in contact recently with someone who has returned from abroad). However, if the disease spreads rapidly, border quarantines have been loose, and physical distancing has not been enforced, contact tracing becomes much harder and public health tracers become overwhelmed. Thus, policies to limit the speed of the spread of the disease have significant implications on being able to trace a larger percentage of contacts, which in turn can reduce the future spread of the disease. When the number of new cases falls and physical distancing guidelines are generally followed, it becomes easier to trace the contacts of new cases. Many countries have had major problems with contact tracing, including the United Kingdom[31] and the United States, but a few — especially Japan, South Korea, Taiwan, and Vietnam — were quite successful, at least in 2020.[32]

2.7 *Insufficient consideration of data needs, collection, and dissemination*

Good decision-making requires good data, good software, and the rapid dissemination of those data.

To understand how a disease is spreading and who is particularly affected, many kinds of information need to be collected from those who are being tested and those tests need to be linked to those who are admitted to hospital, put in the intensive care unit, and/or die. It is extremely useful if these data are collected on a uniform basis across provinces/ states and countries and rapidly disseminated, not only to public health authorities, but, subject to ensuring personal privacy of those tested, to all researchers. In Canada, a recommendation to ensure that data were

---

[31] Peter Roderick, Alison Macfarlane, and Allyson M. Pollock, "Getting Back on Track: Control of COVID-19 Outbreaks in the Community," Analysis, *The BMJ*, 25 June 2020.

[32] Dyani Lewis, "Why Many Countries Failed at COVID Contact-Tracing — but some got it Right," News Feature, *Nature*, 17 December 2020.

consistent across provinces was not acted upon in a timely manner.[33] In the United States, researchers at *The Atlantic* discovered that data on those tested for the virus did not seem to exist for the country as a whole.[34] As a result, they started the COVID Tracking Project, which was later used by the White House as a data source. In the United Kingdom, the software used to aggregate the data associated with swab tests of the public had not been updated. It was not realized that there was a data limit in the Excel program using the old XLS file format (which in 2007 had been superseded by XLSX), and thus some data were not included in the aggregation, leading to undercounting the number of cases.[35]

While age and location seem to have been almost universally collected, it is not clear whether information such as preexisting medical conditions, type of domicile (single-family house, apartment, or condo), type of work, and race[36] has been collected.[37]

Moreover, data on total deaths by week, by province or state, and cause of death need to be collected and disseminated rapidly so that one can determine whether "excess deaths" — which measure the difference between total deaths and what is the normal death rate for that time of year[38] — are similar to the public health statistics on death from the coronavirus disease. If excess deaths greatly exceed deaths attributed directly to the disease, it may suggest that deaths due to the disease are being undercounted or that the indirect effects of the disease, including through policy reactions to it, are quite significant. At the world level, excess deaths far outstripped deaths directly attributed to COVID-19, leading one to believe that deaths due to the disease were undercounted. Although the

---

[33] Ryan Tumilty, "Report's Lessons Not Learned," *Ottawa Citizen*, May 21, 2020.

[34] Robinson Meyer and Alexis C. Madrigal, "Why the Pandemic Experts Failed," *The Atlantic*, 15 March 2021.

[35] Leo Kelion, "Excel: Why Using Microsoft's Tool Caused COVID-19 Results to be Lost," *BBC News*, 5 October 2020.

[36] Christine Ro, "Coronavirus: Why Some Racial Groups are More Vulnerable," *BBC*, April 20, 2020. https://www.bbc.com/future/article/20200420-coronavirus-why-some-racial-groups-are-more-vulnerable.

[37] Wolfson, *Op. Cit.*

[38] The Economist, "Tracking COVID-19 Excess Deaths Across Countries," May 27, 2020, updated regularly. https://www.economist.com/graphic-detail/coronavirus-excess-deaths-tracker.

largest discrepancies are outside advanced economies, even in countries like Canada, it appears that deaths directly due to COVID-19 were likely undercounted in 2020.[39]

2.8 *Insufficient consideration of other health effects of lockdowns and quarantines*

Consideration of policies needs to take into account that there may be unintended consequences for other things that are important for policymakers.[40]

Policies that deal with lockdowns and quarantines need to take into account that these could (i) have serious effects on mental health and (ii) result in hospitals delaying surgeries for serious health conditions. These could lead not only to extended poor health but also death through either suicide or severe worsening of heart disease and cancer. In the COVID-19 pandemic, it is not clear if there was *ex-ante* consideration of this issue. There was a rise in mental health problems such as anxiety disorder, depressive disorder, and substance abuse,[41] but, perhaps surprisingly, not a rise in suicides.[42] As well, it has been estimated that globally some 28 million operations will have been cancelled or postponed over a peak 12-week period (Nepogodiev and Bhangu, 2020). In many Canadian provinces, almost all non-essential surgeries were delayed from mid-March through May 2020; it was estimated that it would take a year or more before that backlog of Canadian surgeries was cleared. In the United States, just over 40% of adults had delayed or avoided medical care by the middle of 2020 according to a web-based survey.[43]

---

[39] Royal Society of Canada, "Excess All-Cause Mortality During the COVID-19 Epidemic in Canada," An RSC Policy Briefing, June 2021.

[40] Itai Bavli, Brent Sutton, and Sandro Galea, "Harms of Public Health Interventions Against COVID-19 must not be Ignored," Analysis, *The BMJ*, 2 November 2020.

[41] Nirmita Panchal, Rabah Kamal, Cynthia Cox, and Rachel Garfield, "The Implications of COVID-19 for Mental Health and Substance Use," *KFF*, 10 February 2021.

[42] Jane Pirkis, Ann John, Sangsoo Shin, *et al.* "Suicide Trends in the Early Months of the COVID-19 Pandemic: An Interrupted Time-Series Analysis of Preliminary Data from 21 Countries," *The Lancet Psychiatry*, 13 April 2021.

[43] Mark E. Czeisler, Kristy Marynak, Kristie E.N. Clarke *et al.*, "Delay or Avoidance of Medical Care Because of COVID-19-Related Concerns — United States, June 2020. *Weekly*, Centers for Disease Control and Prevention, 11 September 2020.

Further unintended health consequences of the lockdowns and other policies include the following: (iii) a decline in routine vaccinations for children, which could lead to increased disease and deaths in the future;[44] (iv) a delay in tuberculosis and HIV treatments in developing countries,[45] which could lead to earlier deaths; (v) overly restrictive birth policies leading to mother stress which could have effects on their baby's health later in life;[46] and (vi) the emphasis on the protection of hospitals leading to worsening crises in long-term care facilities.[47]

2.9 *Insufficient consideration of communication of various messages*

Communication of policy can have significant effects on the effectiveness of policy. Even worse, poor communication can lead to unintended consequences.

In pandemics, there is a difference between communicating "stay at home" or "only go out to exercise and buy essentials, while physically distancing." In the COVID-19 pandemic, there have been differences across countries and regions in the "lockdown" or "stay at home" policies that have been put into place, but even within the same policy, there have been different ways that those policies have been communicated. Initially, in Canada, the message was "stay at home" instead of "stay at home *except* to get daily outdoor exercise, while keeping 2 meters apart, and it

---

[44] Carly Weeks, "Doctors Report Decline in Routine Child Vaccinations," *The Globe and Mail*, May 21, 2020. https://www.theglobeandmail.com/canada/article-doctors-across-canada-seeing-a-drop-in-number-of-routine-child/.

[45] Geoffrey York, "The COVID-19 Pandemic could be 'Devastating' for Battles Against Tuberculosis, HIV and Malaria," *The Globe and Mail*, May 22, 2020. https://www.theglobeandmail.com/world/article-the-covid-19-pandemic-could-be-devastating-for-battles-against/.

[46] Michael Unger and Suzanne King, "Will Pandemic Babies Live with the Effects of their Mothers' Stress," *The Globe and Mail*, May 19, 2020. https://www.theglobeandmail.com/opinion/article-will-pandemic-babies-live-with-the-effects-of-their-mothers-stress/.

[47] Kelly Grant and Tu Thanh Hu, "How Shoring Up Hospitals for COVID-19 Contributed to Canada's Long-Term Care Crisis," *The Globe and Mail*, updated May 21, 2020. https://www.theglobeandmail.com/canada/article-how-shoring-up-hospitals-for-covid-19-contributed-to-canadas-long/.

is okay to talk to neighbors at a distance." Communicating a policy in a way that minimizes the importance of exercise and mental health has serious drawbacks, although the shock and simplicity value of "stay at home" message may be useful for the first few days of a lockdown policy so that the new recommendations are taken seriously by the general public. Continuing to play on fears in the longer run can reduce respect for the authorities and lead to public resentment or, in extremis, civil unrest. There are difficult trade-offs in communication policies that many governments have not handled well.

2.10 *Insufficient consideration of communicable diseases in particular workplaces*

Policies need to take into account particular situations that need to be dealt with explicitly.

Health authorities should know how to prevent the spread of communicable diseases in health facilities. COVID-19 shows that they also need to take into account *ex-ante* that there are particular types of workplaces that are likely to exacerbate the transmission of contagious diseases: Therefore, authorities should introduce regulations to reduce that risk. These include meat and poultry processing plants,[48] distribution centers such as Amazon (in the United States and Canada),[49] and perhaps especially workplaces that have not passed other types of health inspections in the past.

2.11 *Advanced warning systems not up to the task*

There are some crises or disasters for which there can be advanced warning systems. Such is the case, for example, for tsunamis.

---

[48] Justine Hunter, "COVID-19 Puts Unsafe Working Conditions at Meat-Processing Plants," *The Globe and Mail*, May 17, 2020. https://www.theglobeandmail.com/canada/british-columbia/article-covid-outbreaks-shine-light-on-meat-production-in-canada/; and Centers for Disease Control and Prevention (2020a).

[49] Reuters Staff, "Factbox: Coronavirus Cases Reported at 19 of Amazon's U.S. Warehouses," *Reuters*, 31 March 2020; and Tom Blackwell, "More than 400 COVID-19 Cases at Amazon Warehouses in Ontario Amid Concern Over Industrial Spread of Virus," *National Post*, 18 December 2020.

Pandemics, by definition, start in one country and spread to many others. Thus, the identification that there is a new disease that has the potential to spread can be very useful for a number of reasons, including containing the spread, beginning to gear up to counter the pandemic using previously formulated plans, and starting work on developing treatments and vaccines. In Canada, the Global Public Health Intelligence Network was put into place to gather intelligence and to find pandemics early. It worked very well for many years. However, its foreign intelligence operation was effectively shuttered in May 2019 as priorities within the Public Health Agency of Canada shifted to more domestic issues and away from foreign threats, reflecting the priorities of senior officials in the Agency.[50] Many personnel were reassigned to other work in the Agency. As a result, Canada was not on top of the situation as it had been in other outbreaks of disease internationally.[51] It was not the only country in which close monitoring of disease outbreaks was downgraded and/or ignored over the years.[52]

3. Shortcomings in Government Preparation for Pandemics

Although many Western governments had run pandemic exercises and had reports detailing lessons from previous epidemics, the COVID-19 epidemic showed only too clearly their lack of preparation and detailed playbooks as the crisis intensified. Far too often, governments appeared to be struggling to formulate appropriate responses to the crisis. Furthermore, the exercises and reports appeared to be too narrow in only considering medical preparation, ignoring the wide range of government policy

---

[50] See Grant Robertson, "'Without Early Warning You can't have Early Response': How Canada's World-Class Pandemic Alert System Failed," *The Globe and Mail*, July 25, 2020 (updated July 28, 2020). https://www.theglobeandmail.com/canada/article-without-early-warning-you-cant-have-early-response-how-canadas/.

[51] See the July 2021 review, https://www.canada.ca/content/dam/phacaspc/documents/corporate/mandate/about-agency/external-advisory-bodies/list/independent-review-global-public-health-intelligence-network/final-report/final-report-en.pdf.

[52] See Betsy McKay and Phred Dvorak, "Why was No One Ready for Coronavirus?" *The Wall Street Journal*, August 14, 2020.

responses that could be required and their related costs, particularly the possible heavy economic and financial costs of a range of lockdown policies.

As far as we can discern from public sources, countries did not prepare for the economic, financial, and fiscal impacts of the response to the crisis. The direct costs of medical assistance and preparation for the infected are relatively small in relation to national budgets. But, the more stringent quarantine and lockdown policies have had significant implications for national economies, unemployment, financial sectors, and fiscal policies. The impact of these changes on national policies has been magnified by international long-term lockdown policies that have induced major reductions in international trade, travel, migration, and tourism.

In this section, we examine the shortcomings in government preparation for pandemics, including the following: poor oversight and financial implementation of public health plans, lack of preparation regarding the economics of lockdowns, lack of preparation of designs for fiscal policies — such as income supports, job protection subsidies, and loans to firms — that might be necessary in a pandemic, and lack of preparation for the effects of the pandemic on low-income individuals and families, racialized groups, and front-line workers.

3.1 *Poor oversight and implementation of financing of plans*

In the first instance, it is the government under the direction of the executive branch (or cabinet) that is responsible for the oversight of the health department and public health authorities. The government should be ensuring that there are plans and that those plans are being implemented. As noted in Section 2, it is clear that quite often plans were not being implemented. In some cases, this may well have been because the government did not allocate sufficient finance to provide the human resources to implement that plan or to provide for the purchase of equipment and supplies, the expansion of hospitals and the provision of back-up sites, the hiring of sufficient health sector professionals, and the regulation, supervision, and upgrading of long-term care facilities.

In Chapter 4, we return to the question of governance as it relates to pandemic preparation. Suffice it to say that much of the accountability has to lie with the executive branch, but there is also a major role for the legislature.

3.2 *Poor preparation for lockdown design*

Prior to the pandemic, there appears to have been no preparation for or analysis of the following:

(i) Which industries should be considered to be "essential" and how that relates to the input/output structure of the economy,

(ii) The private sector implications and costs associated with various types of lockdown policies and how they might be translated through the economy given its input/output structure,

(iii) The dependence of economic costs on the duration of the lockdowns,

(iv) Major declines in trade, tourism, international supply chains, migration, and international investment stemming from a variety of national lockdowns and border policies of varying severity and longevity around the world,

(v) The effects of real sector output declines on asset markets, financial markets, and credit markets.

3.3 *Lack of preparation for design of relevant fiscal policies*

When there are very large declines in output and employment, the government needs to be prepared to go well beyond the stabilization that comes from the automatic stabilizers — importantly including unemployment insurance — and the stabilization from the reactions of monetary policy, such as that which occurs under flexible exchange rates with inflation targeting. These overarching policies are of three major types: income support programs, protection of jobs and other subsidies to businesses, and loans to businesses. Unfortunately, there is little evidence that most governments had in place options for program design and appropriate procedures and software to implement, at short notice, those programs judged to be among the most efficient and effective.

Income support programs during a pandemic may be needed to help the unemployed, the ill, and the families of children who are ill or whose day care or school is closed because of a lockdown, outbreak of disease, or shortage of staff. Alternatively, the income support could come through some version of the basic income program or through a base payment to every adult earning less than a given amount of money in the previous year. When there is no advanced preparation, programs typically have to be put into place using the foundations provided by unemployment insurance or the personal tax system. These improvised programs will have inefficiencies and be open to fraudulent practices.

An alternative or, more likely, a complement to income support programs is a job protection program that provides subsidies to businesses to pay workers for firms whose revenues have fallen because of lockdowns or because of fears and concerns of the public. Other subsidies or support programs to businesses should be explored in detail, so that they could be implemented in a future pandemic.[53]

If there has not been planning in advance for income support, job protection, and loan programs, then their relative efficiency and effectiveness will not have been closely studied and rushed decisions will have to be made during the pandemic itself.

Because pandemic surprises present an out-of-the-ordinary combination of supply and demand shocks to economic output, fiscal authorities and central banks need to be prepared to not only act quickly to provide economic stimulus but also not be too slow to withdraw stimulus if demand rebounds swiftly relative to underlying supply at some point. By mid-2021, the United States saw a surge in prices as the economy began to recover: Given the extremely large fiscal and monetary stimulus, fears of higher inflation increased. Whether this surge in prices was a short-term reaction or heralds longer-term inflation, only time will tell.

---

[53] One possible solution is to expand catastrophe insurance, with the inclusion of an explicit *ex-ante* government backstop. This is a complex topic, discussed in detail in Crean and Milne (2022).

3.4 *Lack of preparation in considering those groups who might be hit disproportionately*

Low-income and poorly educated people, single-parent families, ethnic minorities, and those with chronic poor health are much more likely to be affected by pandemics than other groups in the population. This is because they are more likely to become unemployed, see declines in their income, to become ill from the disease, to experience worse symptoms if they become ill, and/or to be less well informed about the effectiveness and availability of various protective measures — including vaccination when they become available. All this argues for taking these groups explicitly into account when considering the design of income support and government communication programs. It appears that awareness of these issues only became recognized by governments as the pandemic evolved.

The health of front-line workers (health care and related workers) is another high-risk group, especially if they overlap with any of the groups listed in the above paragraph. This should be taken explicitly into account in policy and communication design.

Experience from previous pandemics was taken into account in dealing with some groups. For example, in Canada, much thought went into the special needs of indigenous groups, given their higher rates of death in previous pandemics and their lower average state of health generally compared with the overall population. However, much less thought went into the potential health and income problems for other ethnic or racial groups until questions began to be asked about their health outcomes. Such policies should draw upon the latest information and analysis from regional, national, and international experience.

4. Shortcomings in Learnings from the First Wave and in Preparing for Vaccines

Many of the shortcomings in preparation for the pandemic became apparent within the first few months. Another shortcoming was the requirement for having a system in place to learn from the experience of other countries (especially those ahead of one's own country in the wave) and earlier waves in one's own country. It was crucial that this analysis be clearly articulated and communicated to policymakers. In addition, one needed to learn from what was happening in the development of new vaccines, especially those based on the relatively new mRNA technology.

4.1 *Learning during the pandemic: Other countries' experience and one's own*

Rapidly developing academic literature on all aspects of the pandemic has been produced since the beginning of the pandemic. This has allowed academics, epidemiologists, physicians, and public health experts to learn from the experience of other countries and from studies comparing experiences across countries.

However, it is not clear if the implications of such studies were always well understood by decision-makers. For example, the implications of aerosol spread of the disease for masking, distancing, and the difference between being close to one another indoors and outdoors were not always evident in the decisions taken.

Another area where policymakers did not appear to learn from experience in other countries — or their own — is in the timing of the adoption of tighter lockdown-type policies. Since typically rising cases precede increasing hospitalizations (including in ICUs), which precede rising deaths, policies aimed at controlling the level of hospitalizations, the utilization of ICUs, and deaths should be based on forecasts. Waiting to tighten policies for various social reasons can be inconsistent with such goals.[54]

4.2 *The ordering of vaccines and portfolio diversification*

By August 2020, it was becoming evident that vaccines for COVID-19 might be developed and ready for use far faster than those for other diseases in the past. Moreover, this could mean that they could be available

---

[54] For example, in the Canadian province of Ontario, a lockdown was delayed until after a holiday weekend.

as early as the first half of 2021. As a result, some countries (especially advanced economies) began to order vaccines for dates starting early 2021. The United States and United Kingdom, where vaccines were actively being developed, typically ordered those vaccines.

Other countries, such as Canada and Australia, where there was little large-scale vaccine development underway, were left to order from producers in other countries. Canada's strategy differed from most countries in the total number of vaccines ordered and its "portfolio diversification" across a significant number of vaccines under development. The Australian Federal government placed two orders, one for a domestic developer and one for Astra Zeneca, for the first half of 2021. The domestic development looked promising, but had some serious deficiencies. In late 2020, the government attempted to order other vaccines, but delivery was delayed. By the middle of 2021, the country was lagging significantly behind other advanced economies in the percentage of its population that had been vaccinated.

It is not clear if pre-pandemic planning in many countries included strategies for obtaining vaccines quickly. In any event, the speed at which the vaccines were developed would have been a surprise to most countries. Some countries reacted quickly to this new information, while others were slow to respond.

There are risks that some vaccines will never be approved, some will be approved well before others, some vaccines will be more effective than others, and some producers with approved vaccines will fail to produce enough to meet their contracted delivery dates. Diversification across potential vaccine suppliers is the optimal policy. Both the United States and Canada incorporated significant diversification into their purchases, which allowed them not only to have administered an average of just under 1.0 dose of vaccine per person by the middle of 2021[55] but also to have bought significant quantities of the two most effective vaccines (Pfizer and Moderna). The United Kingdom had also administered an average of around 1.15 doses of vaccine per person by mid-2021, but this was heavily concentrated in AstraZeneca, which was not quite as effective

---

[55] Our World in Data (2021), "COVID-19 Vaccine Doses Administered per 100 People" data for June 30, 2021.

as the two vaccines most purchased by the United States and Canada in the first half of 2021.

Although it had been flagged by the WHO in 2020, in the spring of 2021, it was becoming increasingly evident that advanced economies were running a huge risk by not making vaccines available to low-income countries and not increasing production of vaccines fast enough. The risk was both medical and economic: The longer a pandemic is out of control in any part of the world, the greater the chance that more deadly variants of the disease will develop and spread to other parts of the world, and the longer the pandemic is affecting a large part of the world's population, the longer it will dampen the world demand and supply of goods and services. The pledge of the G7 countries in Spring 2021 to supply one billion doses of vaccine was quite small relative to the magnitude of the problem.

5. Construction and Use of Models

Models are essential for understanding policy and making predictions, but they are always simplifications of the real world. Indeed, severe oversimplifications can lead to poor forecasts and inappropriate policies. Modelers of contagious diseases face three major challenges that are not faced in other modeling domains. First, each disease has some unique elements in which the disease differs from previous diseases: This information is only revealed by the data over the course of the pandemic. Second, people will change their behavior in response to information regarding cases, severe cases, and deaths — in the home, locally, nationally, and internationally. This behavior will occur even in the absence of changes in public health policy. Third, people will change their behavior in response to public health restrictions on their behavior (e.g., masking, hand washing, distancing, and various forms of lockdowns).

In this section, we discuss the difficulties in modeling methodology, the need to incorporate certain heterogeneities in models to obtain good forecasts, and the importance of providing accurate and nuanced advice. The development of heterogeneous models, prior to the recent pandemic, could have been used to examine overall net economic and social costs associated with governmental policy responses. We recognize that pandemic modeling will always be very difficult, especially for models designed specifically for forecasting many weeks into the future.

5.1 *Fundamental uncertainties in estimating and calibrating models*

A major difference between forecasting pandemics and other phenomenon (such as economic crises or depressions) is that there are no leading indicators that there will be a new disease in the near future. Indeed, it may take a while to identify that there actually is a new disease. Subsequently, one must identify the exact nature of the virus, develop a test for the virus, and prepare test kits so that one can collect data. All this could take several weeks. In the interim, all that is available are data on deaths from the new disease, and these may be underreported, as they could be attributed to pneumonia or some other condition.

It will take time to identify lags that are inherent in the nature of the virus. Those lags, which could differ significantly across viruses, include the following:

- From infection to showing symptoms;
- From primary infection to being infectious to others;
- From showing symptoms to time hospitalized (for those who are eventually hospitalized);
- From showing symptoms to time of death (for those who eventually die);
- From showing symptoms to recovery(for survivors); and
- From showing symptoms to time one is no longer infectious to others.

The greater the variance in these lags, the greater the possible importance of heterogeneities (across age, comorbidities, sex, ethnicity, socioeconomic class, and location) in affecting these lags. The lower the rate of testing, the longer it will be before there are decent estimates of some of these lags.

Prior to having decent estimates, modelers will typically calibrate some of the parameters in their models to earlier diseases, which may or may not have close similarities to the current disease. That said, most models for prediction are a variant of the SIR model (for Susceptible,

Infectious, Recovered) which, in its very simplest form, has only two parameters (requiring data at least on S and I and their rates of change).

Furthermore, even several months after the first detected case, there may be important elements affecting its transmission that are unclear. For example, even in August 2020, there was much uncertainty regarding the epidemiological characteristics of COVID-19: the percentage of people contracting the disease who remain asymptomatic,[56] the length of time that people getting the disease remain immune (Alberta Health Services, 2020), how the "viral load" affects transmission (including severity of the disease and probability of dying),[57] and whether there are certain conditions under which people have partial immunity to the disease before ever contracting the disease.[58] All these uncertainties greatly increase the uncertainty of forecasts regarding the hospitalization and death numbers to be expected from the disease. In turn, this affects advice regarding the optimal policies to be put into place. Forecasting is not the only reason we have models, however. Knowing very little about many of the parameters of a mathematical model does not mean that models of viral behavior have no important insights about appropriate health preparations and low-cost policies to implement almost immediately — such as handwashing, masking, and physical distancing wherever possible.

5.2 *Important heterogeneities*

There are three important types of heterogeneities that are relevant for modeling the spread of a contagious disease: (1) locations within a given geographic area, (2) the geographic location, and (3) characteristics of the population.

---

[56] Roz Plater, "As Many as 80 Percent of People with COVID-19 Aren't Aware They Have the Virus," *Healthline*, May 28, 2020, https://www.healthline.com/health-news/50-percent-of-people-with-covid19-not-aware-have-virus.

[57] Ananya Mandal, "Does High COVID-19 Viral Load Mean More Risk of Infection?" *News Medical Life Sciences*, April 21, 2020, https://www.news-medical.net/news/20200421/Does-high-COVID-19-viral-load-mean-more-risk-of-infection.aspx.

[58] Freddie Sayers, "Karl Friston: Up to 80% Not Even Susceptible to COVID-19," report on an interview with Karl Friston, UnHerd, June 4, 2020, https://unherd.com/2020/06/karl-friston-up-to-80-not-even-susceptible-to-covid-19/.

Because the spread of contagious diseases depends on close contact with others, one can look at the probabilities of close contact within a geographic area by workplace, residence, place of leisure, and type of transportation. In the current pandemic, there is much evidence that rates of infection have been much higher at specific places. Some workplaces by their very nature — many of them involving "line" work — lead to workers being very close to one another. In the current pandemic, this has been very evident in meat and poultry processing plants (Centers for Disease Control and Prevention, 2020a) and distribution centers, as mentioned in Section 2. Residences involving close proximity also lead to greater possibilities of disease transmission. Such locations would include prisons in Canada (Correctional Service Canada, 2020) and the United States, migrant worker dormitories (migrant agricultural workers in Canada and migrant workers in Singapore),[59] crowded housing of low-income families, and some apartment buildings. Then, there are residences that involve close contact with workers, especially medical personnel and personal support workers, such as long-term care facilities, seniors' residences, hospitals, and group homes. As noted earlier in this chapter, this risk can be more dangerous when workers are employed at more than one of these locations. Places of leisure, involving large numbers of people, would include spectator sporting facilities, beaches, concerts, conventions, religious services (Centers for Disease Control and Prevention, 2020b), funerals[60] and weddings, theaters, and cinemas. Local transport by subway or light rapid transit is suspected of having increased infection rates in large cities such as New York, but buses and taxis also could have similar effects.

Any of these places of close contact with large numbers of people are potential "super-spreading locations," as long as many of those frequenting

---

[59] Michael Bociurkiw, "An Infection Surge has Exposed Singapore's Migrant-Worker Blind Spot," *The Globe and Mail*, May 15, 2020, https://www.theglobeandmail.com/opinion/article-a-covid-19-surge-has-exposed-singapores-migrant-worker-blind-spot/.

[60] See, for example, Holly McKenzie-Sutter, "Anxiety Lingers as N.L. Officials Trace Bulk of COVID-19 Cases to Funeral Home", The Canadian Press, *National Post*, April 5, 2020, https://amp.flipboard.com/@NowYouKnow/anxiety-lingers-as-n-l-officials-trace-bulk-of-COVID-19-cases-to-funeral-home/a-5JsqARHdTuOdMX5EO5rX2w%3Aa%3A220507260-ef119214bf%2Fnationalpost.com.

these locations also have contacts in other locations. (Those with many such contacts are known as "super spreaders.") The existence of such locations opens the potential for surges in the number of cases and deaths, as well as making modeling very difficult. On the other hand, without knowing details, one can implement a policy to minimize the probability that super-spreading will occur in such locations. Thus, closing places of leisure has been one of the earliest steps taken in earlier pandemics (such as the "Spanish flu" of 1918–1919)[61] and was one of the earliest steps taken in the current pandemic. Large gatherings of any kind and super-spreading locations need to be a focus of policy right from the beginning.

In the very early period of modeling a pandemic in a given country or region, a lack of data means that many of the parameters will have to be taken from the behavior of disease spread in other countries. However, one needs to recognize that geographic location in itself is a source of heterogeneity, because of varying population density, the percentage of commuters who use public transport, the degree of contact with those who have recently travelled abroad or are visiting from abroad (especially from countries where the disease is pronounced), cultural norms (such as the normal degree of social distancing and the use of masks when ill),[62] and the average characteristics of the population.

Characteristics of individuals, such as age, sex, preexisting medical conditions, and ethnicity, can have pronounced effects on their death rates and even their likelihood of infection. The relative death rates by age of those infected can be very different across contagious diseases. Typical influenza epidemics most affect the old and very young. However, the Spanish flu had very large death rates for those in their twenties and thirties. The COVID-19 pandemic has had extremely low death rates for those under 40 years, with increasing rates for older people, especially for those in their seventies, eighties, and nineties.

Heterogeneities can also arise from differing abilities of medical facilities to handle a surge in cases (thus potentially affecting death rates),

---

[61] Jones, E. W. (2007).

[62] Lin and Meissner (2020) show that countries or U.S. cities that had higher mortality to the Spanish flu in 1918 were more likely to have higher initial mortality in the COVID-19 pandemic.

the dosage of exposure ("viral load"), and potentially from multiple strains of a virus (Avery *et al.,* 2020).

In terms of prediction models within a given region or country, the heterogeneities that are the most important are likely differences across subpopulations i in the mean number of people (R_{0i}) that an infected person will infect directly at a time when everyone is susceptible. This is inextricably linked with the subpopulations inhabiting or frequenting the "super-spreading locations" discussed above. Thus, for example, health care workers and personal support workers who do not have the proper personal protective equipment are likely to have a higher R_{0i} than retired persons living in their own home, physically distancing, and wearing masks in crowded places. The implementation of good health policies (e.g., handwashing, physical distancing, mask wearing, the wearing of personal protective equipment by health and other personnel), as well as various versions of quarantine or lockdown policies, can reduce the effective R_{0i}'s of subpopulations. Expanded SIR models that incorporate heterogeneities across people, which focus on subpopulations with different R_{0i}, have very different implications both for forecasting and policy as compared to the simple SIR model (Ellison, 2020). The implications of such models include the following:

- It might take a long time to have a good understanding of the dynamics of a pandemic.
- It might be very difficult ex post to obtain good estimates of the health, social, and economic effects of lockdown policies and reopenings.[63]
- Herd immunity effects may slow a pandemic's spread at levels of prevalence in the overall population lower than the simplest SIR models would predict.

---

[63] This is a highly contentious and complex research agenda that is still evolving. Issue one: the health effectiveness in the short and long run of a strong lockdown or a series of lockdowns. For an analysis based on US state data, see https://www.nber.org/system/files/working_papers/w28930/w28930.pdf.

A second issue is the cost–benefit analysis of lockdowns taking into account health, social, and economic consequences of lockdowns. For a critical survey, see https://www.sfu.ca/~allen/LockdownReport.pdf.

For another viewpoint on the cost and benefits of lockdowns, see The Economist, "How to Assess the Costs and Benefits of Lockdowns," 3 July 2021. https://www.economist.com/finance-and-economics/2021/07/01/how-to-assess-the-costs-and-benefits-of-lockdowns.

- Keeping high-contact subpopulations (high R_{0i}) from contracting the disease can be extremely important in reducing the spread of the disease. (This argues for more preparation in regard to the super-spreading locations mentioned in the early part of this sub-section.)
- Judicious use of lockdowns could be more effective in cutting total deaths from the virus over the full length of the pandemic than simple SIR models would claim. These benefits should be balanced against increased deaths from late diagnosis from other serious illnesses.
- Keeping policies that eliminate activities that cause high spread rates would be important (this could include forbidding certain inside activities without wearing masks and forbidding large gatherings).

In many jurisdictions, it is not clear if prior to the current pandemic the authorities had in place a suite of models, some of which could have been, with some tweaking, helpful for understanding the spread of the virus. That suite of models should have included models with heterogeneities important for understanding some of the key features of the dynamics of previous epidemics or pandemics, such as the Spanish flu, SARS, MERS, and 2009 H1N1 flu.

5.3 *Modeling economic, overall health, and social effects of pandemics*

Although there were a number of models designed to explain and predict infection and deaths from pandemics prior to COVID-19, these were generally not integrated into models of the economic, overall health, and social effects of pandemics. The optimal social policy to combat a pandemic is not the one that minimizes deaths from the pandemic. Rather, it needs to take into account the overall welfare of the population, which would be a function of overall deaths and health, social, and economic well-being, now and in the future.[64]

---

[64] The social and economic dynamics are important. Many Western countries have run up huge government debts. Education has been severely disrupted, with detrimental long-run impacts on students, especially the poor and disadvantaged. Both of these are likely to have effects on national economic welfare in future years.

The concept of "excess deaths" tries to estimate the marginal impact on deaths of both the virus and the various policies that have been put into place to combat the virus. It captures the effects on death of worsened mental health, delays in seeking medical attention, delays in non-critical surgeries, a worsened economy, changes in stress levels, potentially lower levels of other communicable diseases, lower traffic accidents, and potentially other factors as well. Most of these factors would affect overall health and social well-being as well as deaths.

Social well-being is also affected by restrictions in freedom of movement and opportunities to participate in certain prohibited social private and public events.

After the current pandemic was well underway, there were many useful models created to explore some of the effect on both deaths and consumption (or GDP) of various policies (including doing nothing). These models examine effects on overall welfare of the population as a whole or various groups within that population. Most of the theoretical core of these models depends heavily on key properties of the current pandemic, such as a very high percentage of the deaths in the population occurring among older people, a group that has very low labor force participation. Thus, without significant tweaking, the models may not be useful for future pandemics whose features could be very different. Nonetheless, they point to some key elements that may be useful in models of future pandemics that would capture economic, overall health, and social effects: age groups, labor force participation by age group, and employment in industries deemed "essential" or "non-essential."[65] As these elements, as well as the effects of different R_{0i}'s across key subpopulations, were also important in the Spanish flu, it is unfortunate that no one tried to calibrate a model for that pandemic in one or more countries, trying to mimic some of its key features. That would have provided some insights into places to start modeling far earlier in the current pandemic, even though, as mentioned earlier, the Spanish flu differed markedly from COVID-19 in the

---

[65] The following papers examine policies and their effects on both the economy and health in the context of models that contain one or more of the key heterogeneities mentioned in the text: Glover *et al.* (2020); Rampini (2020); Aum, Lee, and Shin (2020); Acemoglu *et al.* (2020).

age groups that suffered high death rates. Thus, COVID-19 requires different policies to deal with subpopulations most at risk. Spanish flu was quite lethal for a much younger working population than is the case for COVID-19. But, this observation regarding age groups must be tempered by recognizing other important demographic factors (such as poverty and crowded living conditions) when formulating a policy response.

6. Concluding Comments

The lack of preparedness for the COVID-19 pandemic, which became evident within only a few months after the WHO declaration of the pandemic, resulted from four major types of shortcomings. First, even when there were problems noted in previous epidemics, clear plans were not put in place to deal with similar situations. Second, there was a lack of transparency prior to the pandemic about plans and preparation. Third, it was not clear if authorities had considered *ex-ante* the effects of pandemic policies on overall health (including mental health). Fourth, governments were largely unprepared to consider the interdependence of health, social, and economic factors in a pandemic and how appropriate "lockdown," income transfer, and loan policies could be implemented in practice. These shortcomings have increased the economic, health, and social costs of the pandemic.

Another weakness of the policy response during the pandemic arose from insufficient learning by policymakers from both the first wave and from what was happening internationally. Even though a few countries were becoming aware by August 2020 that vaccines might be ready for general use by the end of the year, many countries neglected to order vaccines in time and to have a diversified portfolio of contracts with vaccine makers. The portfolio strategy was most effective given the uncertainty over which vaccines would be approved, which vaccines would be most effective, and which vaccine producers would be able to meet their time commitments for production and delivery.

Because pandemics can be so different in their health consequences, models have a very limited role for policymaking early in a pandemic. However, to be most useful later in a pandemic, they need to incorporate important heterogeneities across age groups and types of location.

Importantly, to be useful in examining which policies might be best, they need to incorporate not only the way the disease spreads but also the interdependent effects on overall health and the economy.

Overall, a vast majority of governments and public health authorities in advanced economies have performed poorly in preparing for the pandemic. In this respect, this is similar to the failures of a majority of financial regulators and supervisors prior to the global financial crisis. There are many direct parallels between the weaknesses in preparation for COVID-19 and those in preparation for the financial crisis. We turn our attention to these parallels in Chapter 3.

References

Acemoglu, D., Chernozhukov, V., Werning, I. and Whinston, M. D. (2020). "Optimal Targeted Lockdowns in a Multigroup SIR Model," NBER Working Paper 27102, May. https://www.nber.org/papers/w27102.

Alberta Health Services (2020). "Topic: Can People with Previous COVID-19 Infection become Re-infected by the SARS-CoV-2virus?" Updated May 12. https://www.albertahealthservices.ca/assets/info/ppih/if-ppih-COVID-19-reinfection-rapid-review.pdf.

Aum, S., Yoon (Tim) Lee, S. and Shin, Y. (2020). "Inequality of Fear and Self-Quarantine: Is There a Trade-off between GDP and Public Health?" NBER Working Paper 27100, May. https://www.nber.org/papers/w27100.

Avery, C., Bossert, W., Clark, A., Ellison, G. and Ellison, S. F. (2020). "Policy Implications of Models of the Spread of Coronavirus: Perspectives and Opportunities for Economists," NBER Working Paper 27007, April. https://www.nber.org/papers/w27007.pdf.

Bell Canada (2020). "Bell Acquires 1.5 Million Protective Face Masks to Support Frontline Healthcare and Other Essential Public Workers Throughout Canada," Press release, April 17. https://www.bce.ca/news-and-media/releases/show/bell-acquires-1-5-million-protective-face-masks-to-support-frontline-healthcare-and-other-essential-public-workers-throughout-canada-1.

Centers for Disease Control and Prevention (2020a). "COVID-19 Among Workers in Meat and Poultry Processing Facilities — 19 States April 2020," *Morbidity and Mortality Weekly Report*, May 8 (posted online May 1). https://www.cdc.gov/mmwr/volumes/69/wr/mm6918e3.htm.

Centers for Disease Control and Prevention (2020b). "High COVID-19 Attack Rate Among Attendees at Events at a Church — Arkansas, March 2020," *Morbidity and Mortality Weekly Report*, May 22 publication (posted online May 19). https://www.cdc.gov/mmwr/volumes/69/wr/mm6920e2.htm.

Correctional Services Canada (2020). "Inmate COVID-19 Testing in Federal Correctional Institutions June 11, 2020" and other dates. Accessed June 12, 2020. https://www.csc-scc.gc.ca/001/006/001006-1014-en.shtml.

Crean, J. and Milne, F. (2022). "Covid and Other Catastrophes — Systemic Risks Neglected by Financial System Reform," Working Paper forthcoming.

Dijkema, B. and Wolfert, J. (2019). "People Over Paperwork," Cardus, November 12. https://www.cardus.ca/research/work-economics/reports/people-over-paperwork/.

Ellison, G. (2020). "Implications of Heterogeneous SIR Models for Analyses of COVID-19," NBER Working Paper 27373, June. https://www.nber.org/papers/w27373.pdf.

Jones, E.W. (2007). *Influenza 1918: Disease, Death, and Struggle in Winnipeg*. Toronto: University of Toronto Press.

Glover, A., Heathcote, J., Krueger, D. and Ríos-Rull, J.-V. (2020). "Controlling a Pandemic," NBER Working Paper 27046. http://www.nber.org/papers/w27046.

Johns Hopkins Coronavirus Resource Center (2020). "All State Comparison of Testing Efforts," Johns Hopkins Coronavirus Resource Center, May 28, 2020, updated daily. https://coronavirus.jhu.edu/testing/states-comparison.

Jones, E. W. (2007). *Influenza 1918: Disease, Death, and Struggle in Winnipeg*. Toronto: University of Toronto Press.

Lin, P. and Meissner, C. (2020). "Note on the Long-Run Persistence of Public Health Outcomes in Pandemics," NBER Working Paper No. 27119, May. https://www.nber.org/papers/w27119.pdf.

Nepogodiev, D. and Bhangu, A. (2020). "Elective Surgery Cancellations due to the COVID-19 Pandemic: Global Predictive Modelling to Inform Surgical Recovery Plans." *British Journal of Surgery*, May 12. https://bjssjournals.onlinelibrary.wiley.com/doi/full/10.1002/bjs.11746.

Office of the Provincial Health Officer, British Columbia (2020). "Order of the Provincial Health Officer to Licensees of Long-term Care Facilities and Private Hospitals," March 27. https://www2.gov.bc.ca/assets/gov/health/about-bc-s-health-care-system/office-of-the-provincial-health-officer/reports-publications/COVID-19-pho-order-movement-health-care-staff.pdf.

Our World in Data (2020). "How Many Tests are Performed Each Day?" May 28, 2020, updated daily. https://ourworldindata.org/coronavirus-testing.

Rampini, A. (2020). "Sequential Lifting of COVID-19 Interventions with Population Heterogeneity," NBER Working Paper 27063, April. https://www.nber.org/papers/w27063.pdf.

The Ottawa Hospital (2020). "Ottawa's First COVID-19 Assessment Centre Opens Today," Press release, undated (about March 13). https://www.ottawa hospital.on.ca/en/newsroom/ottawas-first-COVID-19-assessment-centre-opens-today/.

Working Group on Long-Term Care (2020). "Restoring Trust: COVID-19 and The Future of Long-Term Care," A Policy Briefing, Royal Society of Canada, June. https://rsc-src.ca/sites/default/files/LTC%20PB%20%2B%20ES_EN.pdf.

Chapter 3

Parallels

1. Introduction

In Chapter 2, we described substantial weaknesses in the preparation by public health authorities and governments for the COVID-19 pandemic. These weaknesses increased the health and economic costs of the pandemic relative to what they would have been if pre-existing recommendations had been followed and a wider set of plans and procedures had been put into place. There are a number of striking parallels between these weaknesses and the weaknesses in financial system regulation prior to the Global Financial Crisis (GFC) of 2008–2009. No doubt there are other areas in terms of preparation for crises or natural disasters where there are similar parallels. All this argues for sharing experiences across fields which, at first glance, may seem unrelated.

In Section 2, we discuss 10 parallels between the lack of preparation by financial system regulators prior to the GFC and the lack of preparation by public health authorities and governments prior to COVID-19. In each case, we start with a description of the lack of preparation by financial system regulators, followed by a parallel weakness in COVID-19 preparation. The 10 weaknesses that we consider concern the following:

1. Insufficient requirements for stocks (of capital and liquidity or equipment) as well as for their replenishment
2. Insufficient public disclosure of data consistent across entities regarding risks

3. Insufficient advance planning regarding various "lender-of-last-resort" facilities
4. Insufficient stress testing required by the authorities, including using historically stressful periods
5. Insufficient attention given to warning signs that trouble was on the way
6. Lack of appreciation of possible contagion from abroad
7. Lack of appreciation of certain operational risks, including those related to weaknesses in corporate culture
8. Lack of appreciation that appropriate regulation and planning needed to take a system-wide approach, including effects on the real economy and the interconnectedness of stresses
9. Lack of appreciation that models for looking at effects on the real economy need to incorporate heterogeneity of individuals or groups
10. Lack of appreciation of the effects of a crisis on unregulated or less-regulated entities

We note in advance that some of the illustrations of weaknesses, whether in the GFC or the pandemic, are actually examples of more than one weakness.

In Section 3, we consider the steps that were taken to deal with each of the deficiencies in financial system regulation following the GFC, and the parallel steps that now need to be taken to deal with the deficiencies in pandemic planning.

2. Lack of Preparation

The size and variety of problems encountered during the GFC in many advanced economies showed that financial regulators, especially bank regulators, and the institutions they regulated were not prepared to deal with substantial shocks. Five of the areas where there was a lack of preparation were where there were insufficient requirements, public disclosure, advance planning, stress testing, or attention to warnings. The other five areas were associated with lack of appreciation of what could go wrong or how problems could spread. Each of these 10 areas had parallels in lack of preparation for COVID-19. In this section, we discuss the 10 areas where there was lack of preparation by financial regulators (and their regulated institutions) and the parallels in public health authorities and governments. In each subsection, we denote part (a) for the deficiency in the financial sector area and part (b) for the parallel COVID-19 deficiency.

2.1 *Capital and liquidity requirements*

(a) Banking regulators and other financial system prudential regulators are required to regulate the safety and soundness of financial institutions (and sometimes of the financial system as a whole). Thus, they are concerned with the solvency and liquidity of these institutions, which are often interrelated.

In good times at a financial institution, unexpected losses on some loans and other assets plus reserves for future expected losses plus payments on deposits and liabilities are more than offset by earnings on other loans and assets. However, when the economy weakens, unexpected losses and reserves for future expected losses can be so large that profits become negative, thus eating into bank equity capital. Therefore, prior to the GFC, bank regulators choose to impose requirements on bank equity capital, either in relation to risk-weighted assets as in Basel I[1] and Basel II of the Basel Committee on Banking Supervision (2006) or overall assets (termed a "leverage ratio"), so as to increase the likelihood that the institutions will remain solvent. During the GFC, it became evident that the amount of capital that was required for many institutions in a number of countries was insufficient to prevent them from approaching insolvency, thus leading to government bailouts. Some countries that required higher capital than the international Basel standard performed better than those that did not.[2] Also, some countries went farther than Basel by adding a requirement for a leverage ratio.[3]

---

[1] See "Basel I: the Basel Capital Accord" in "History of the Basel Committee," https://www.bis.org/bcbs/history.htm.

[2] For example, Canada had a higher required risk-weighted capital ratio, as well as requirements for higher quality Tier 1 equity capital (Longworth, 2014, p. 92).

[3] This was true of Canada, as well as for U.S. commercial banks (Longworth, 2014, p. 93).

Despite the fact that there were clear capital requirements, it was not quite clear what was expected of banks as their level of capital declined significantly (i) while still remaining above the requirement, (ii) while falling somewhat below the requirement and (iii) while approaching zero.

Perhaps surprisingly, given the importance of banking liquidity, there were no international standards for banks on either the requirements for bank liquidity plans or liquidity ratios prior to the GFC, although in 2008 there was significant discussion about what liquidity plans should contain (Basel Committee on Banking Supervision, 2008a, 2008b). Many individual jurisdictions, did, however, require some types of liquidity planning and did have at least notional requirements for the holding of liquid assets. For example, U.S. banking regulators have long had a CAMELS rating system for banks, where the "L" stands for liquidity (or asset liability management).

(b) There are some interesting parallels between these weaknesses in regulation and planning, and the weaknesses in the preparation of public health authorities for pandemics in the period prior to COVID-19. First, although there were typically numerical targets for appropriate stores of personal protective equipment, ventilators, and other equipment, it was not clear what was to happen when the amount of equipment that had not reached its expiry date fell below the requirement. Second, it was not always clear what the targets should be as a ratio of, for example, population. Third, it was not clear that all relevant senior policy makers in public health authorities and governments understood the existing plans for stores of equipment. Finally, the detail in which plans were made for expanding intensive care units, the number of hospital beds, and the number of nurses when a pandemic struck is not clear. Some jurisdictions appeared to have a limited understanding of the risks associated with running hospitals beyond their normal capacity for extended periods of time even in "good times."

2.2 *Insufficient public disclosure of comparable data on risks and lack of timeliness of data*

(a) At the time of the GFC, banks in many jurisdictions had to disclose some key aggregate balance sheet data on a monthly and/or quarterly basis, as well as earnings data on a quarterly basis. However, they typically did not have to disclose much industrial and geographic data on their loans, nor did they have to disclose direct data on their credit and markets risks by industry or geographical region, taking into account their full balance sheet as well as off-balance-sheet exposures. Differences in national accounting standards[4] and regulatory reporting standards meant that these measures were often not consistent across countries, although the data were consistent within countries and some data were roughly comparable internationally.

Although some simple liquidity ratios could be calculated from the monthly balance sheet data, in many jurisdictions, banks were not required to calculate their daily liquidity positions by currency (and thus be able to report them immediately to their regulators). In some cases, the lags in daily liquidity position calculation could extend to a week. Also, it was hard for some international banks to know what their liquidity positions were for the bank as a whole. These were both very problematic during the GFC.

(b) Data disclosure problems also became very evident early in the COVID-19 pandemic as problems that were generally well known before the pandemic had never been remedied. These data problems had strong parallels with the data problems that were evident in the financial system during the GFC. First, some of the data that should have been collected from those tested for COVID-19 (such as race, age, and comorbidity) were not collected from day one. Second, often the data that were collected were not stored in comparable ways across jurisdictions (e.g., in Canada across provinces and in the European Union across countries), and thus it was difficult to do comparative studies. Third, reporting systems had not been constructed in such a way that all data collected on-site at a hospital, testing center, or laboratory on a given day could be aggregated by the following morning, meaning that there was a lack of

---

[4] Although International Financial Reporting Standards (IFRS) issued by the International Accounting Standards Board (IASB) were first adopted in 2004 by many countries and subsequently by many more, the U.S. Financial Accounting Standards Board (FASB) still issues its own Generally Accepted Accounting Principles (GAAP). Although there has been convergence between these two sets of standards in some areas, there are other areas where there has been no significant convergence.

timeliness in data. Fourth, lack of timeliness in reporting deaths from all causes, disaggregated by cause, meant that it was difficult to know the number of deaths indirectly resulting from the pandemic (e.g., more deaths from cancers and heart problems, fewer deaths from car accidents, and fewer or more suicides). Fifth, differences in defining what it means to die from or with COVID-19 (rather than from another condition that led the person to be in the hospital in the first place or from complications from COVID-19 such as breathing problems) made it difficult to interpret COVID-19 death data across jurisdictions. Thus, it was difficult to study what actions were most effective in reducing deaths when the data on deaths were not comparable.

2.3 *Insufficient planning regarding lender-of-last-resort facilities*

(a) Prior to the GFC, central banks had informal statements of their lender-of-last-resort facilities for banks and similar financial institutions, or even more formal "policies" (such as Bank of Canada, 2004; Daniel, Engert, and Maclean 2004–2005). These were typically "narrow" in scope, considering loans to individual financial institutions (on a standing or extraordinary basis) or repo facilities (either standing or on a regular auction basis) available to a group of institutions (primary dealers in government debt, or banks and other deposit-taking institutions). They were generally designed to deal with funding liquidity of institutions and not generalized market liquidity problems. The experiences from the market problems in the asset-backed commercial paper market in August 2007 and through the GFC made it clear that careful research and preparation for generalized market liquidity problems would have been helpful in the crisis.

(b) Jurisdictions where multiple governance levels store health-related equipment to be used in pandemics (federal government, provincial/state governments, regional health authorities, and individual hospitals and other health facilities) need to have a clear understanding of which level is responsible for maintaining these stores and under what circumstances the equipment will be lent or given (by the health equipment "lender of last resort") to lower levels of authorities. For example, in Canada, it is not clear that such an understanding existed prior to the COVID-19 pandemic.

2.4 *Insufficient stress testing required by authorities*

(a) Prior to the GFC, bank regulators and central banks had begun to require individual commercial banks to carry out regular stress tests, as well as to participate in system-wide stress tests on an annual, biennial, or less frequent basis. As part of their five-year Financial System Assessment Program (FSAP) reviews for advanced countries, the IMF required a system-wide stress test in which it played an important part in the design of the stress tests to be carried out. Unfortunately, the two largest countries in the world, the United States and China, did not agree to have FSAPs until after the GFC (Longworth, 2014, p. 95). In addition, the stresses assumed for market liquidity were not large enough to capture the extreme liquidity events in the GFC.

To make matters worse, the required value-at-risk calculations for the calculation of bank capital were typically based on very short time periods and did not include historically stressful periods. The period before the GFC had been dubbed "The Great Moderation" because of its lower variability in GDP growth and price inflation, an expression that also captured the regulatory complacency of that period.

(b) In the case of pandemic planning, there had been significant studies in various countries about what had been learned from the SARS epidemic and the Ebola crisis, as we discuss further in Chapter 4. Unfortunately, much of what was discovered was ignored in terms of ongoing pandemic preparation. Furthermore, there is little evidence of frequent use of stress testing and wargames (especially using large stresses relative to a long span of history (e.g., using the Spanish flu pandemic of 1918–1919) and taking into account new scientific information on diseases passing from other animals to humans.

2.5 *Insufficient attention given to warning signs*

(a) Through the 1990s and early 2000s, there was growing evidence from academic and policy institution sources that rapid credit growth, especially against a background of growing asset price increases, was associated with a heightened probability of a financial crisis (Kaminsky and Reinhardt, 1999; Borio and Lowe, 2002; Rajan, 2005). It was evident that some innovations in mortgages in the United States (sub-prime mortgages, Alt-A mortgages, no-downpayment mortgages, and low rates on the first few years of a mortgage) had led to a sizeable increase in the supply of residential mortgages and that house prices had peaked in 2006 and were starting to decline. Although the Federal Reserve understood that there were risks associated with these developments, they (i) downplayed them because they felt that financial institutions were well capitalized, and (ii) even if there were a very sizeable decline in housing prices, the direct exposure of financial institutions to mortgage loans was not large relative to that capital. Unfortunately, this glossed over the indirect exposure of financial institutions (especially investment banks not directly supervised by the Federal Reserve) to the housing market and mortgages through securitized mortgages and derivative products. Given the warning signs, it is clear *ex post* that the Fed had not been prepared to entertain scenarios where bank capital was inadequate relative to the potential deleterious effects of indirect exposures, including potential market illiquidity and funding illiquidity.

(b) In the first two months of the COVID-19 pandemic, the WHO and national health authorities did not give enough attention to the warning signs from early reports of what was happening in China and to the early spread out from China to other countries. Canada had effectively gutted its early warning group, the Global Public Health Intelligence Network, in May 2019 and so was unable to properly evaluate the little that Canada was hearing. The WHO established the Independent Panel for Pandemic Preparedness and Response in 2020 to report in May 2021 to, among other things, ensure that the WHO would in the future address threats to health effectively.

2.6 *Lack of appreciation of possible contagion from abroad*

(a) Because national financial systems are highly integrated internationally, national credit losses and related liquidity events flow across countries. During the GFC, credit losses associated with the U.S. real estate market were transmitted to other institutions around the world, which held financial instruments whose payoffs reflected the real estate losses.

In addition, large international financial institutions are linked by interbank financial transactions, and in the case of the very largest institutions, subsidiaries operate across national borders. These connections can allow losses and fear of losses in a jurisdiction to cross borders and appear in another country's financial system.[5]

Finally, given the international nature of finance, risky lending practices were copied in other countries to a greater or lesser extent. Within the U.S., less prudent financial institutions were bankrupted (or bailed out), while more prudent institutions survived. Ireland also had a major real estate boom, loose lending, weak bank supervision and a major banking crisis. Conversely, in Canada, the large commercial banks with strong risk management traditions and with strict regulatory supervision survived the GFC.

(b) When the virus appeared in Wuhan, the Chinese government prevaricated in informing other nations. The WHO was also implicated in not providing sufficient warning to countries around the world. As the virus spread to Europe and the U.S., lack of governmental preparation added to the spread of the disease and an increasing death rate. In contrast, because of better preparation, geographic isolation and other factors, some countries were better able to contain or reduce the impact of the virus. For example, South Korea, Japan and Taiwan had experience with previous viruses emanating from China and had preventative measures in place. In particular, these countries can only be entered by sea or air, so that timely introduction of effective quarantine measures, testing and contact tracing contained the spread of the virus. To be effective, quarantine and other procedures require careful monitoring and professional training of staff. Quarantine periods require careful monitoring: more virulent strains of a virus may require more demanding quarantine. Conversely, a virus may mutate into a more benign strain and require less demanding quarantine procedures.

---

[5] See IMF (2008). Although this international contagion occurred during the GFC, earlier financial crises had similar impacts.

Australia provides another example that is instructive in terms of both strong and weak preparation. The Australian federal government, with the cooperation of the states, introduced very restrictive travel arrangements whereby travellers arriving in Australia were quarantined in supervised hotels. The quarantine system was arranged and supervised by the military, with one exception — the state of Victoria, which chose a private contractor. Unfortunately, the behavior of this contractor led to a breakdown in the Victorian quarantine system as we discuss further in Chapter 4.

A further complication arose due to many countries outsourcing their supplies of PPE, vaccines and other products critical to combating the virus. With international supply chains disrupted and countries at the manufacturing source of the supply chain hoarding supplies, severe shortages appeared. Similar supply chain problems have occurred for other imported commodities. Lockdown and quarantine restrictions have disrupted some international supplies and the provision of services internationally.

A good example of disruption of services has been the lack of planning and risk management associated with an event that led to a major contraction in the number of foreign students entering tertiary education in many Western countries. In the case of Australia, large universities were funded by up to 40% from foreign fee-paying students. After the pandemic started, exacerbated by the associated severe restrictions on incoming flights, the Australian universities suffered a major decline in funding, leading to significant layoffs of academic staff.

2.7 *Lack of appreciation of certain operational risks, including those related to weaknesses in corporate culture and governance*

(a) The GFC revealed major problems in the analysis of mortgage credit. Credit risks were estimated by models calibrated by past data. The model predictions during 2002–2006, in the great moderation period, had forecasted manageable credit risks on securitized mortgages. The mathematical/computer model predictions lulled financial markets and regulators into a false sense of security surrounding the system of writing and packaging high-risk mortgages. There were economists, regulators and bankers who were only too well aware of the dangers[6] associated with underwriting these high-risk mortgages and their packaging into securitized tranches, but in too many cases they were ignored. The problem was exacerbated by fraudulent and reckless lending and misleading selling of the securitized products to naïve investors. When U.S. house prices plateaued and then declined in 2006–2007, the credit risks rose quickly catching many bankers, regulators and investors unaware. Investment banks and commercial banks with large investment and trading operations were heavily exposed to securitized mortgages. Investment banks, who had been in the securitization chain, found few buyers for their securitized mortgage products, as their securitized investor market dried up. They were faced with very large inventories of risky assets with rapidly declining valuations. Investment bank insolvency (and fears of insolvency) created a panic that led to an international financial and economic recession only partially moderated by massive bank bailouts by the U.S. and European governments.

Although fraud was an element in creating the GFC, a more common failing was corporate myopia and complacency. These failings were reinforced by compensation packages for CEOs, senior executives, and traders that gave incentives to emphasize short-term results (profits — not adjusted for risk — and "sales"/new business) over long-term risk-adjusted profits. There were many instances where companies had CEOs and Boards who ignored the warnings of competent risk managers. Complacency and arrogance were not just isolated in private financial institutions but also amplified by the mainstream media in reporting to the public, and worst of all, by poor preparation of a number of financial and bank regulatory systems around the world. Too many regulators relied on "box-ticking" as opposed to looking at some of the major underlying

---

[6]The models suffered two major risks: model risk and estimation risk. Model risk occurs when the models omit risks, especially severe infrequent downside events. Estimation risk occurs because model parameters are estimated with error, and in the worst situation, can be very biased when based on periods with asset booms. For a discussion in the context of the GFC, see Milne (2009).

risks. The Basel I bank regulatory framework, which was extremely simplistic, was still being used in some jurisdictions. The more comprehensive Basel II framework was just starting to be used in other jurisdictions.

(b) A parallel in lack of government preparation in operational risk areas has been revealed by the COVID-19 pandemic. It became clear in 2020 that many governments had been complacent and ill prepared for a pandemic. There were serious weaknesses of oversight in the governance of long-term care homes. Other examples were the Canadian government having effectively dismantled an important pandemic warning organization, as noted above, and Canada having no capacity to produce vaccines, so that it had to rely on foreign suppliers for vaccines.

These examples demonstrate serious failures of governance in not responding to previous reports warning of the stresses that a pandemic would impose on key sectors. In turn, these stressed sectors would have serious flow-on effects on other sectors of the society, health system and the economy.

For many jurisdictions, there were failures in not developing sophisticated media and communication policies in explaining to the public the uncertainties concerning the virulence and lethality of the virus, and the various strategy options that could be chosen by policy makers. As policy makers introduced new restrictions, they often appeared panicked and inconsistent, leading to increasing scepticism of their competence. Few policy makers explained conditional strategies based on a constant inflow of new or more reliable data.

2.8 *Lack of appreciation that appropriate regulation and planning needed to take a system-wide approach including effects on the real economy and the interconnectedness of stresses*

(a) One of the major lessons learned from the GFC was the importance of regulation and planning, especially when considering system-wide implications of major credit events across national and international real and financial markets. Warning signs were there for all to see in the rapid increase in U.S. real estate debt over the 2002–2007 period. The credit boom was concentrated in various geographic locations in the U.S., with high credit risk characteristics and credible reports of poor credit under-writing standards, e.g., No Income, No Job, no Assets (NINJA) loans. These high-risk loans were concentrated in the temporary inventory of a small number of large investment banks operating in the shadow banking sector.[7] This sector, though very important in the financial system, was lightly regulated. Most of the models used by the public and private sectors did not take into account the systemic nature of the risks. Given the network of interbank/institution exposures, losses would be magnified by fears of contagion and further losses. Financial disruption, wealth losses and unemployment would impact other real sectors of the economy, especially through demand for durable products.

U.S. regulators faced serious gaps and overlaps in responsibility and supervision. The investment banks, which had been acting as conduits for the securitized mortgage market, were regulated by the Securities and Exchange Commission (SEC), not by any of the federal banking regulators for commercial banks. The SEC had little expertise in the prudential regulation of credit risks. Because of these regulatory gaps, the crisis caught the U.S. government unprepared. Indeed, the Federal Reserve seemed to be unaware of the serious systemic risks over the first year of the crisis. The Lehman Brothers bankruptcy and resulting panic ended that complacency. No one U.S. institution had been charged with looking at overall financial system stability, and there were overlaps in the very complicated banking regulatory structure, with both federal and state regulators. At the federal level alone, there were five financial industry regulators: the Federal Reserve System, the Federal Deposit Insurance Corporation, the Office of the Comptroller of the Currency, the National Credit Union Administration, and the Office of Thrift Supervision (which, in 2011, had its oversight functions merged with the OCC).

Because international financial markets are so connected, weaknesses in regulatory oversight and supervision spill over into other national

---

[7]The temporary inventories were required for packaging loans into securitized debt. When the crisis hit in mid-2007, the market for these securitized loans dried up and the investment banks were left holding this inventory of bad loans.

financial systems. For example, the Greek financial system became seriously impaired, but many of the losses appeared on bank balance sheets in other countries (e.g., French and German banks).

(b) The parallels in the experience with the pandemic are striking. Many countries in the West had not prepared for the systemic impacts of pandemics and associated policy responses. Their public health regulators were slow to analyze the lethality and virulence of the virus, especially its serious consequences for the elderly and/or people with comorbidities. Long-term care home supervision in many jurisdictions was perfunctory and ineffective: the consequences were deadly. This was compounded by the shortages of PPE and other supplies.

Analysis and preparation for pandemics should consider broader consequences than purely medical issues relating to quarantine, tracing, and various versions of lockdowns. For example, planning and exercises prior to the pandemic appear to have ignored broader health, economic, social and fiscal consequences of major, lengthy lockdown policies. Some of the economic costs could be ameliorated by various government subsidy schemes. The costs of these schemes would imply dramatic increases in private and government borrowing. Better pandemic preparation would have introduced protocols and systems to ensure that financial support was used as effectively as possible.

Part of pandemic preparation would include plans for a balanced political dialogue with the populace about policy options and their consequences. As a pandemic is socially and economically stressful, it is critical that communication be clear and honest, with revised policies carefully explained.

2.9 *Lack of appreciation that models for looking at effects on the real economy need to incorporate heterogeneity of individuals or groups*

(a) Major financial crises usually originate in the following: credit supply shocks that affect a subset of real sectors (where they often go hand in hand with asset bubbles), major increases in environmental risks (e.g., tsunamis, earthquakes, pandemics), trade disputes or major wars. The costs are not borne equally across the economy: some households and sectors are hard hit, while others prosper. The ability of households to buffer shocks will depend importantly on shocks to their income and wealth, as well as the sectors in which they work; there are important differences across income and wealth deciles. Thus, heterogeneities in microeconomic behavior, as well as financial-real linkages, need to be taken into account by macroeconomic authorities, financial regulators, and the financial institutions themselves.

Prior to the GFC, macroeconomic theories and models used by most central banks relied largely on overly aggregated theories of the economy with primitive additions to deal with financial markets.[8] Macroeconomics used aggregates for consumption, investment and GDP.

Many risk managers in financial institutions and their regulators did not take a microeconomic (sectoral) view of credit risk, nor did they appreciate the many feedback mechanisms between the real and financial sectors.

Given the microeconomic factors at work, policy frameworks that just concentrate on macroaggregates will miss the critical causes and triggers of an economic/financial crisis. This theoretical (and related empirical) analysis creates blindness in prudential preparation, and when a financial crisis hits, lack of preparation leads to inappropriate policy implementation with major excess costs. For example, blanket programs could be introduced, which miss the critical microeconomic differences across sectors and their behavioral responses.

(b) The outbreak of the COVID-19 pandemic caught most jurisdictions unprepared. In particular, policy makers largely relied on models that did not sufficiently discriminate across demographic and geographic characteristics. The Imperial College macromodel was reported in the media as predicting extremely high death rates for the U.K., leading to panic in the media and pressure on the U.K government to institute widespread lockdowns.[9] But within weeks, COVID-19 statistics demonstrated that deaths were concentrated in the elderly and/or those with

---

[8] Other statistical models were used, but they also had major limitations.

[9] See https://www.nature.com/articles/d41586-020-01003-6.

comorbidities. The virus was contagious but very much less deadly for the younger population, where the virus was often asymptomatic.[10]

2.10 *Lack of appreciation of the effects of a crisis on unregulated or less-regulated entities*

(a) One of the major problems that emerged in the U.S. during the GFC was the often ineffective patchwork regulation of financial institutions. While the FDIC regulated deposit-taking commercial banks, the SEC regulated investment banks. The large investment banks played a key role in distributing securitized mortgages. When the U.S. housing market turned down and mortgage defaults mounted, the less prudent investment banks (Bear Sterns, Lehman Brothers), and a major insurance company (AIG) writing default insurance were exposed to huge losses. Given the highly integrated interbank market, these losses threatened to bring down much of the financial system in the U.S. and the Western world.

A major problem was the SEC and prominent government advisors' inability to understand the risks taken by the investment banks and associated financial institutions. Many financial innovations were introduced outside the institutions regulated by the commercial bank regulators. One of the reasons that securitized credit expanded so rapidly in the 2000–2006 period was its ability to avoid prudential regulation imposed on commercial banks.

One of the downsides in no regulator taking a system-wide approach to the financial sector was a lack of realization that other financial institutions that had close relationships with banks would be hard hit by the weaknesses elsewhere in the financial sector, especially the banking sector and financial markets. In the GFC, this showed up in a few ways. One example was that finance companies, even those whose assets were sound, were unable to raise funds easily from parent banks or in the commercial paper market. As a result, their credit-granting abilities diminished.

---

[10]For a discussion of the complexities of modeling a new virus in a pandemic model and the media's role in focusing on worst-case outcomes, see https://insights.som.yale.edu/insights/in-defense-of-mathematical-models.

A second example is that hedge funds were often unable to carry out the types of transactions with banks that they were used to doing, such as securities borrowing. As a result, they could not contribute to market liquidity.

Since the crisis, U.S. investment banks have been supervised under the prudential regulatory system. But there is always an incentive for risky lending to find ways to avoid prudential regulation. A major policy issue is to anticipate these incentives and devise methods for reducing systemic risks, so that institutions bear the costs of their risk-taking and do not benefit from bail-out subsidies.

(b) Similar regulatory problems occurred in the pandemic. In many jurisdictions, ongoing poor supervision of long-term care homes left residents to die in appalling conditions. As there were no regulatory restrictions against the practice, staff often worked across a number of homes, increasing the risks of cross-infection. Other jurisdictions acted more promptly, requiring stringent protection of the aged and careful supervision of carers. Clearly good regulatory and supervisory practices that may have been regarded as overzealous in normal times paid off in the pandemic.

3. Steps to Deal with Deficiencies

Even before the GFC was over, international standards setters, such as the Basel Committee on Banking Supervision (BCBS) and the Financial Stability Board (formerly Financial Stability Forum) and domestic financial regulators, began taking steps to deal with the deficiencies that had been noted. The large government bailouts that had taken place during the crisis and the significant effects on the real economy both heightened the need for such steps. Over several years, the deficiencies in the 10 areas we noted in Section 2 were dealt with in one way or the other by regulators. The BCBS initially was looking at a major revision to Basel II, but as it became more and more evident that a larger number of fundamental changes were required, the changes were packaged as Basel III (Basel Committee on Banking Supervision, 2017) and the Basel Framework (Basel Committee on Banking Supervision, 2021). In the following sections, the steps to deal with these 10 deficiencies are described together with their parallels in what should be required in planning and preparing for future pandemics.

3.1 *"Capital and liquidity"*

(a) In Basel III, the definition of capital was improved and the required amounts of capital (including by more appropriately calculating some of the risks that the capital was supposed to cover) were raised. Also, international banks were required to meet both a risk-weighted capital requirement and a leverage requirement, and a countercyclical capital requirement was added. Banks are now required to have recovery plans which would enable them to restore their viability — including having sufficient capital — relatively quickly. These plans must be updated regularly and assessed by domestic regulators.

Basel III also introduced two liquidity standards: the liquidity coverage ratio to deal with short-term liquidity problems and the net stable funding ratio to deal with the funding of longer-term assets (Basel Committee on Banking Supervision, 2013, 2014). Domestic regulators[11] also require banks to have liquidity plans.

(b) In addition to having requirements for the stocks of personal protective equipment, ventilators, and other equipment (which likely already existed in most jurisdictions), there needs to be "recovery planning" for the replacement of equipment when it reaches its expiry date. Also, the required stocks of such equipment should rise with the population as well as with the share of the population that is most likely to be more susceptible to serious problems from pandemics, such as those with comorbidities, the elderly, and perhaps infants as well. Just as in the case of capital requirements, the actual stocks of equipment relative to requirements need to be reported to the most senior policy makers (including cabinet ministers) and reviewed and evaluated by a designated agency, as described in more detail in Chapter 4.

---

[11] For example, the Office of the Superintendent of Financial Institutions (2020) in Canada, the Bank of England in the U.K., and the Australian Prudential and Regulatory Authority.

Intensive Care Units (ICU), hospital beds, and nurses are somewhat like "liquidity" in the sense that either their numbers can be raised or they can be reallocated to areas set aside for pandemic patients. A clear "liquidity plan" is, however, needed in advance, one that would specify in detail how overall ICUs, beds and nurses could be increased at short notice and the implications of reallocating these resources to pandemic patients on the health of those waiting for surgeries or treatments.

3.2 *Insufficient public disclosure of comparable data on risks and lack of timeliness of data*

(a) By the very end of the GFC, large banks were typically able to produce their liquidity positions daily. Required liquidity plans of banks have to include how a bank will "actively monitor and control risk exposures and funding needs" (Basel Committee on Banking Supervision, 2008b). Disclosure of more disaggregated balance sheet data and key risks on a uniform basis across international banks is now required as part of pillar 3 of Basel III. The principles of the new requirements of pillar 3 are that disclosures should be clear, comprehensive, meaningful to users, consistent over time, and comparable across banks (Basel Committee on Banking Supervision, 2015, paras 12 and 13).

(b) Uniformity of detailed data collection in a timely manner needs to be given high priority and included in pandemic planning. The principles of pillar 3 would seem to be applicable.

Jurisdictions need to be in a position from day one of a potential pandemic to collect important detailed data on those tested, those admitted to the hospital with the disease, and those who die of the disease. These should include, but not be limited to, the following: race, age, occupation, address, and comorbidities. In countries with provincial/state or regional health authorities, these data need to have common definitions and be easily collected and shared in systems that can produce reports in a timely manner. Timeliness should mean that all data collected on a given day, whether at a hospital, testing center, or laboratory, should be available to be aggregated the following morning.

Data on deaths from all causes in all jurisdictions should be collected and made available in a timely manner so that indirect effects of the pandemic on deaths by cause can be readily known. In addition, there needs to be the active use of a uniform definition of what it means to die from a pandemic disease.

3.3 *Insufficient planning regarding lender-of-last-resort facilities*

(a) The experience of the design and use of lender-of-last-resort facilities during the GFC led to some central banks writing about the principles regarding such facilities. For example, the Bank of Canada wrote and spoke about such principles (Engert, Selody and Wilkins 2009; Longworth 2010). Subsequently, this led the Bank of Canada to describe its ongoing facilities (Bank of Canada, 2020).[12] Although this did not cover all the facilities used during the market liquidity problems at the beginning of the COVID-19 pandemic, the descriptions of both the ongoing facilities and the principles surely guided the Bank's behavior.

More generally, central banks reviewed the lessons from their overall experience with lender-of-last-resort facilities during the GFC, as evidenced by the workshop held by the Bank for International Settlements Monetary and Economic Department (2014)[13] for central bankers and academics. The areas discussed included the stigma of drawing on facilities, the pros and cons of transparency (especially about individual institutions), moral hazard, governance and international dimensions of the lender-of-last-resort role.[14]

(b) In countries with multiple health jurisdictions, there needs to be a clear understanding of which jurisdictions are ultimately responsible for providing health equipment, which levels are going to acquire and store

---

[12] See also https://www.bankofcanada.ca/markets/market-operations-liquidity-provision/ framework-market-operations-liquidity-provision/emergency-lending-assistance/ and https://www.bankofcanada.ca/markets/market-operations-liquidity-provision/ framework-market-operations-liquidity-provision/#providing-liquidity.

[13] See https://www.bis.org/publ/bppdf/bispap79.pdf.

[14] See Li, Milne and Qiu (2021) for a theoretical discussion of various subtle policy issues.

equipment for lower jurisdictional levels, and which principles and rules are going to guide the way in which such stores will be made available. Such principles and rules should be made public.

3.4 *Insufficient stress testing required by authorities*

(a) Stress testing took on a much more important role following the GFC. Central banks constructed models that could be used to carry out top-down stress testing,[15] and both bottom-up and top-down testing were used. Stress tests were used by banks in their capital planning exercises and U.S. regulatory authorities put much emphasis on the results of their prescribed stress tests in the capital requirements for the banks under their supervision (Federal Reserve Board, 2020).[16] Historically stressful periods were used as one input into the size of stresses, and they were required to be used in value-at-risk calculations related to capital requirements.

(b) Stress testing and wargames should be used in pandemic planning at regional, provincial/state, and especially national levels. They would also be useful at an international level. Chapter 5 describes how these would be helpful after post mortems of the COVID-19 pandemic are held and new pandemic plans are put into place.

3.5 *Insufficient attention given to warning signs*

(a) Since the GFC, there has been much more attention to warning signs and financial system weaknesses. The analysis done by the Financial Stability Board Standing Committee on Assessment of Vulnerabilities, by the International Monetary Fund (in its *Global Financial Stability Report*), and by various central banks in their financial stability reports has become much more sophisticated and wide-ranging. As part of this effort, there

---

[15] These include the Risk Assessment Model of Systemic Institutions (RAMSI) model at the Bank of England (Burrows, Learmonth and McKeown, 2012) and the MacroFinancial Risk Assessment Framework (MFRAF) at the Bank of Canada (Gauthier, He and Souissi, 2004; Fique, 2017).

[16] See https://www.federalreserve.gov/publications/files/2020-dec-stress-test-results-20201218.pdf.

has been more attention paid to credit, especially household credit — and within that to residential mortgage credit, as a longer-run leading indicator of financial crises and economic downturns (Borio and Drehmann, 2009; Gourinchas and Obstfeld, 2012; Schularick and Taylor, 2012; Mian, Sufi and Verner, 2017; Mian and Sufi, 2018; and Krishnamurthy and Muir, 2020). The role of household debt service ratios as a shorter-run leading indicator has also been noted (Drehmann and Juselius, 2013; Drehmann, Juselius and Korinek, 2018). This attention has been driven largely by research in academia, the Bank for International Settlements, and the International Monetary Fund.

(b) The absence of key groups to look for warning signs of a pandemic on a daily basis has been noted in Canada and the United States, and by the WHO. As a result, such groups will be created or re-established. It is important that these groups be also charged with looking for new types of warning signs.

3.6 *Lack of appreciation of possible contagion from abroad*

(a) Since the GFC, there has been increased cooperation by international financial bodies and central banks to reduce the risks from international contagion.[17] This cooperation, in which the Financial Stability Board has been a major driver, operates at two levels: First, major financial centers have cooperated by introducing what is regarded as best practice prudential supervision of their domestic banking systems. One of the major tools used by regulators for increasing the financial resilience of their banking systems is the use of stress tests, where banks are required to show whether they would be solvent when hit by a major economic downturn. In addition, banks were ordered to increase their equity and liquidity cushions through the use of mandated minimal ratios. If a banking crisis does occur, the Financial Stability Board has developed new procedures for

---

[17] The Financial Stability Board (FSB) and the Bank for International Settlements (BIS) are just two of the several international organizations that sponsor conferences, international meetings, research, etc. to enhance best practice for national and international financial stability.

dealing with weakened Systemically Important Financial Institutions (SIFI's). These include Living Wills, Resolution Procedures and Bail-in Debt to ensure that institutions can continue operating, limiting contagion through interbank markets. Second, international banks operating in different countries are required to carry out national stress tests and participate in IMF FSAP stress tests and to integrate these tests into their risk management practices. Thus, there is international integration and cooperation at the firm *and* regulatory levels.

But the current system is not perfect: there will be other feedback from domestic banks and non-banks that will interact with the international banks. A further problem is that national stress tests run the danger of being inconsistent across borders, and with international cooperation, there is a danger of groupthink where certain risks are regarded as unimportant: "That event will never happen."

International cooperation is laudable, but there are doubts that in a crisis, cooperation will falter, as national political systems will place their own interests above that of other nations. There are no easy solutions to this problem.

In summary, there has been extensive work trying to reduce the risks from international financial contagion. While the system has become more resilient, it is far from perfect.

(b) There is still much work to be done dealing with pandemic preparedness internationally as well as domestically. At the international level, the WHO has failed on several occasions to inform or coordinate national pandemic policies. There have been failures at three levels: the provision of timely technical advice and information on international infections; international cooperation on international travel restrictions; and the distribution of vaccines. There has been policy confusion over the effectiveness of national responses, taking into account important national differences in demography, the quality and effectiveness of health organizations and national preparedness. It is clear that international cooperation can reduce infection rates through timely testing, quarantine, etc. for international travellers, thus reducing the likelihood of contagion from abroad. Cooperation of the largest countries is required for the WHO to be more effective.

3.7 *Lack of appreciation of certain operational risks, including those related to weaknesses in corporate culture and governance*

(a) Since the GFC, there have been many studies of its causes and discussions of lessons to be learned. Subsequent changes in regulations of financial institutions have been designed to make the system more stable and less likely to be susceptible to a future financial crisis. Model and estimation risk are now better understood. Corporate and executive incentives have been changed to reduce incentives for reckless risk-taking. Regulators have focused on the importance of corporate culture and governance overall within banks.

But shrewd regulators and risk managers are only too well aware that as the memory of the GFC fades, corporate and regulatory complacency can create unrecognized risks in the system. The regulatory system must be anticipatory and prepared. For example, cyber risk is a constant threat to the financial system. Financial institutions have been under attack for years, as hackers and fraudsters have been trying to access information, blackmail the institution, etc. But more disturbing is the growing threat of cyberwarfare, instituted by aggressive states as one component of major political, economic, and social warfare just short of kinetic warfare.[18] This threat to financial stability transcends the usual boundaries of financial supervisory analysis.

(b) The pandemic has revealed extremely serious deficiencies in health planning and preparedness in many countries and jurisdictions. Although there had been pandemic exercises in many countries, they had not incorporated health and non-health consequences of policy responses. For example, the economic, fiscal and social consequences of severe lockdown policies had not been modeled or included in political policy playbooks, as we discuss further in Chapter 5. Even worse, there seemed to have been a casual disregard for a number of the early lessons in the pandemic by senior politicians and bureaucrats. The first pandemic wave in February–April 2020 had revealed the vulnerability of long-term care homes and quarantine hotels to waves of infections due to lax health and

---

[18] Elliott and Jenkinson (2020).

safety regulations. In some jurisdictions, these lessons were not learned, so that unnecessary second wave infections and deaths occurred. The major policy responses after the GFC are an indication of what *should* happen after the COVID-19 pandemic subsides.

3.8 *Lack of appreciation that appropriate regulation and planning needed to take a system-wide approach including effects on the real economy and the interconnectedness of stresses*

(a) Since the crisis, the national financial regulators have been devising systems that attempt to reduce the risks of international and domestic financial contagion and its impact on the rest of the economy. This is a complex process that is necessarily a work in progress.[19] The real and financial systems are closely interlinked, so that regulation and policy responses should take that fact into account.

To illustrate the interconnectedness of the real and financial sectors, consider the evolution of the GFC. It was created by a real estate boom, fueled by poor underwriting in the mortgage market. As the U.S. real estate market declined in 2006–2008, borrowers defaulted, the losses and bankruptcies flowed into defaulting mortgages and into the shadow banking system, where credit risk had been securitized. As the losses flowed through some of the highly exposed financial systems, lending became more cautious. Consumers reduced expenditure on durable goods, firms laid off workers and the recession rippled through both the real and financial sectors.[20]

Since the GFC, financial institutions have been more prudent in lending, restricting exposures to credit risks, both directly and indirectly. The regulatory system is attempting to build in real and financial feedback into their systems.

Also, in jurisdictions such as the United States, the United Kingdom, and the European Union, reforms of the regulatory systems were

---

[19] For example, see the discussion in Haldane (2017).
[20] See Mian and Sufi (2014).

undertaken to centralize the macroprudential oversight of the entire financial system, thus taking a more system-wide perspective.

(b) A similar approach is needed in post-COVID-19 reforms of the medical and pandemic control systems. Prior to the pandemic, planning was narrowly focussed on public health and medical responses without considering the wider impact of policies that could be implemented to combat the pandemic. It is well known that lockdown strategies were controversial, especially given the severity and length of any lockdown policy. If lockdown policies were regarded as feasible in prior planning, then why were the broader health, economic, social consequences and costs not part of the exercises? Policy makers should have been better prepared in understanding collateral medical, social and economic costs when choosing over the portfolio of responses. This is a lesson that should be learned in future preparations, as we discuss further in Chapters 4 and 5.

3.9 *Lack of appreciation that models for looking at effects on the real economy need to incorporate heterogeneity of individuals or groups*

(a) The GFC taught many lessons for regulators and policy makers. One of the lessons was that there is considerable heterogeneity across individuals and firms. Academics and central banks have improved their models by incorporating differences across household behavior that depend on their income, wealth, and indebtedness. These models have also incorporated richer linkages between financial and real sectors. For example, some households and firms were prudent and not directly implicated in highly risky borrowing. Banks were not homogeneous in their lending and risk management practices. Some risky and/or poorly run financial institutions failed, while others survived without any direct government assistance. Indiscriminate government policy responses were financially and fiscally wasteful. But even worse they can create moral hazard in banks' risk management behavior anticipating future financial crises. Regulators and bank supervisors have introduced procedures and regulations to reduce moral hazards and poor policy responses. For example, the widespread use of stress tests, and minimum liquidity and leverage ratios are policies that can be used to force banks to reform poor risk management practices.

There was geographic heterogeneity in the housing bubble and the wave of defaults.[21] For the U.S., this was not only at the state level but extended down to zip codes. Some areas were hard hit, whereas other areas survived with minor losses. These geographic indicators were proxies for homogeneity in credit risk in economically exposed communities. Microdata is a standard source of information in any competent bank credit system.

(b) Early in the pandemic, governments appeared to rely on highly aggregated models with population average transmission and mortality rates. These models exaggerated the impact of the virus in predicting extreme death rates, not taking into account many relevant factors, e.g., individual behavior that reduced infection in vulnerable populations or, at the other extreme, the high risks for residents of long-term care homes.

Within months, more micro-based models were developed, which incorporated important demographic characteristics of the virus. In principle, these predictions provided advice on policies that would be more effective and less costly. For example, the lethality of the virus for the elderly, especially in long-term care homes or in multi-generational households, should have led to concentrated early responses targeting those high-risk demographics; they did in some jurisdictions but not others.

Future viral pandemics may have very different demographic characteristics from the COVID-19 virus. Consequently, the timely collection of microdata and the application of micro-based models based on that data should improve predictive power and allow more targeted policies.

It became clear by late April 2020 from the statistics where some of the more important vulnerabilities lay and the direction that more nuanced policies should take. But many governments blundered in not implementing more effective policies, creating undue deaths and hardship.[22] Policymakers largely relied on models that did not discriminate across demographic and geographic characteristics.

---

[21] See Mian and Sufi (2014).

[22] Around 90% of Australian COVID-19 deaths were located in the state capital, Melbourne. These deaths occurred over a period June–September 2020. The neighboring state, NSW, with similar demographics had a far more effective and responsive health system for dealing with pandemics. By the end of 2020, the NSW death rate was a small fraction of the Victorian death rate.

It is critical that detailed forensic analyses of the pandemic are implemented. The lessons learned should be incorporated in subsequent exercises or wargames.

3.10 *Lack of appreciation of the effects of a crisis on unregulated or less-regulated entities*

(a) During the late 1990s until the crisis, credit was migrating from commercial banks into securitized markets which were lightly regulated in the U.S. In the U.K., similar light-touch regulation allowed some banks to take on high credit risk. The crisis revealed the folly of this approach.

Since the GFC, investment banks have been regulated under the same rules as the deposit-taking commercial banks. Regulation has become more demanding. There have been regular stress tests of the banking system. Banks have far more stringent capital and financial ratios. There is a widespread perception that the banking system is more stable than prior to the GFC.

A problem has arisen where financial risks have migrated to the less regulated sectors. There is a constant battle in regulating and defending the core banking system while monitoring fringe financial institutions: it is critical to create mechanisms to reduce the risk of contagion migrating from the fringe to the core system. But there is always an incentive for risky lending, which is often associated with financial innovations, to find ways to avoid prudential regulation. A major policy issue is to anticipate these incentives and devise methods for reducing systemic risks, so that institutions bear the costs of their risk-taking and do not benefit from bailout subsidies.

(b) From our recent experience with COVID-19, we have seen disturbing parallels. The most obvious has been failures of long-term care regulation in many jurisdictions. There have been too many cases in this area where health and pandemic preparation have been rudimentary. For example, staff have been allowed to work at multiple locations, thus increasing the risk of infection. Some regulatory authorities moved quickly to guard against these risks: the results in terms of reduced infections and deaths were laudatory. The jurisdictions that acted promptly required stringent protection of the aged and careful supervision of carers. Clearly good regulatory and supervisory practices that may have been regarded as overzealous in normal times paid off in the pandemic. Similar precautions prevented quarantine hotels from becoming infections centres. Other jurisdictions had far laxer regulations and weak response mechanisms in place, implying a series of public health disasters.

We assume that there will be policy action to remedy the long-term care problems. But the larger problem is that no pandemic is quite the same, so preparations should be flexible enough to move quickly when the demographic and geographic risks are discerned, so that responses are targeted, effective and commensurate with the risks. At the same time, regulators must be aware of innovations in health care practices undertaken to lower costs which raise the risks to the overall health system of bad outcomes.

Because pandemics and viruses can differ markedly in terms of their impact on different demographics, contingency plans should include strains that attack other demographics. For example, consider a virus (unlike COVID-19) that is far more lethal for children and far milder for adults. The micro response should concentrate on protecting children and may well avoid general societal lockdowns. This would require regulatory bodies to be prepared for such an event, requiring close cooperation of school governance with medical authorities.

4. Conclusion

It was clear by the first half of 2008 that most regulators and many banks had not undertaken enough preparation for the possibility of a financial crisis. However, both internationally and domestically, most of the problems that needed attention were noted in late 2008 and early 2009. It did nonetheless take about 10 years until most of the major regulatory changes, such as some elements of Basel III, were formally adopted and, even now, some regulatory requirements are effectively still tightening as institutions were given a number of years to meet those major changes. Fortunately, even given these lags, the more stringent regulations and better risk management by banks meant that the banks were in relatively good shape to face the shock of COVID-19 in 2020.

By very early in the COVID-19 pandemic, it was clear that public health authorities and governments had not undertaken enough preparation. It turns out that 10 of the areas where there had not been enough preparation had strong parallels with areas where bank regulators and banks had not done enough 12 years earlier. These were the following: stocks of equipment, data collection and sharing, lending facilities, stress testing and wargames, early warning indicators and systems, contagion from abroad, operational risks, a system-wide approach (including effects on the real economy), models incorporating the heterogeneity of individuals, and effects on less-regulated parts of the system.

Some post mortems on what has gone wrong during the pandemic have already begun. These include the study by the Independent Panel for Pandemic Preparedness and Response set up by the WHO, which has a broad remit, down to provincial examinations of what went wrong in long-term care facilities in Ontario and Quebec. It will be important for all 10 areas discussed in this chapter to be examined thoroughly in post mortems. Where appropriate, these need to be done internationally, nationally, provincially, and regionally. Moreover, these examinations should start in 2022 with the aim of having recommendations in early 2023 so that governments and public health authorities can begin to implement new plans soon after memories fade quickly. Thus, one needs to make decisions and act relatively quickly — more quickly than financial regulators did following the GFC.

In Chapter 4, we will flesh out more fully what needs to be done to put together post mortems and plans, as well as the governance of these processes.

References

Bank for International Settlements Monetary and Economic Department (2014). "Re-thinking the Lender of Last Resort," BIS Papers No. 79, September.

Bank of Canada (2004). "Bank of Canada Lender-of-Last Resort Policies," *Financial System Review*, December, pp. 49–55.

Bank of Canada (2020). "Rules Governing Advances to Financial Institutions," 11 August.

Basel Committee on Banking Supervision (2006). "Basel II: International Convergence of Capital Measurement and Capital Standards: A Revised Framework — Comprehensive Version," 30 June.

Basel Committee on Banking Supervision (2008a). "Liquidity Risk Management and Supervisory Challenges," 21 February.

Basel Committee on Banking Supervision (2008b). "Principles for Sound Liquidity Risk Management and Supervision," 25 September.

Basel Committee on Banking Supervision (2013). "Basel III: The Liquidity Coverage Ratio and Liquidity Risk Monitoring Tools," 7 January.

Basel Committee on Banking Supervision (2014). "Basel III: The Net Stable Funding Ratio," 31 October.

Basel Committee on Banking Supervision (2015). "Standards: Revised Pillar 3 Disclosure Requirements," January.

Basel Committee on Banking Supervision (2017). "Basel III: Finalizing Post-crisis Reforms," 7 December.

Borio, C. and Drehmann, M. (2009). "Towards an Operational Framework for Financial Stability: "Fuzzy" Measurement and its Consequences," BIS Working Papers No. 284, June.

Borio, C. and Lowe, P. (2002). "Asset Prices, Financial and Monetary Stability: Exploring the Nexus," BIS Working Papers No. 114, 2 July.

Burrows, O., Learmonth, D. and McKeown, J. (2012). "RAMSI: A Top-down Stress-testing Model," Bank of England Financial Stability Paper No. 17, 11 September.

Daniel, F., Engert, W. and Maclean, D. (2004–2005). "The Bank of Canada as Lender of Last Resort," *Bank of Canada Review*, Winter, 3–16.

Drehmann, M. and Juselius, M. (2013). "Evaluating Early Warning Indicators of Banking Crises: Satisfying Policy Requirements," BIS Working Papers No. 421, August.

Drehmann, M., Juselius, M. and Korinek, A. (2018). "Going with the Flows: New Borrowing, Debt Service, and the Transmission of Credit Booms," NBER Working Paper No. 24549, April.

Elliott, J. and Jenkinson, N. (2020). "Cyber Risk is the New Threat to Financial Stability," IMF Blog. https://blogs.imf.org/2020/12/07/cyber-risk-is-the-new-threat-to-financial-stability/.

Engert, W., Selody, J. and Wilkins, C. (2009). "Financial Market Turmoil and Central Bank Intervention," *Bank of Canada Financial System Review*, June, 71–78.

Federal Reserve Board (2020). "Federal Reserve Board Announces Individual Large Bank Capital Requirements, which will be Effective on October 1," press release, 10 August.

Fique, J. (2017). The Macro Financial Risk Assessment Framework (MFRAF), Version 2.0, Bank of Canada Technical Report No. 111, September.

Gauthier, C., He, Z. and Souissi, M. (2004). "Introducing Funding Liquidity Risk in a Macro Stress-Testing Framework," *International Journal of Central Banking* 10(4), 105–141.

Gourinchas, P.-O. and Obstfeld, M. (2012). "Stories of the Twentieth Century for the Twenty-First," *American Economic Journal: Macroeconomics*, 4(1), January, 226–265.

Haldane, A. (2017). "Rethinking Financial Stability," Speech at 'Rethinking Macroeconomic Policy IV' Conference, Washington, D.C., Peterson Institute for International Economics, 12 October.

Herring, R. and Schuermann, T. (2019). "Objectives and Challenges of Stress Testing," To appear in J. D. Farmer, A. Kleinnijenhuis, T. Schuermann, T. Wetzer (eds.), *Handbook of Financial Stress Testing*, Cambridge University Press.

IMF (2008). Global Financial Stability Report, "Market and Funding Illiquidity: When Private Risk Becomes Public," Chapter 3. World Economic and Financial Surveys (Washington, April).

Kaminsky, G. L. and Reinhart, C. M. (1999). "The Twin Crises: The Causes of Banking and Balance of Payments Problems," *American Economic Review*, 89(3), June, 473–500.

Krishnamurthy, A. and Muir, T. (2020). "How Credit Cycles Across a Financial Crisis," NBER Working Paper No. 23850, revised, September.

Li, M., Milne, F. and Qiu, J. (2021). "Central Bank Screening, Moral Hazard, and the Lender of Last Resort Policy," *Journal of Banking Regulation*, https://doi.org/10.1057/s41261-021-00159-z.

Longworth, D. (2010). "Bank of Canada Liquidity Facilities: Past, Present and Future," Speech given at the C.D. Howe Institute, Toronto, 17 February.

Longworth, D. (2014). "The Global Financial Crisis and Financial Regulation: Canada and the World," in R. Medhora and D. Rowlands, *Crisis and Reform: Canada and the International Financial System*, Canada Among Nations 2014, Centre for International Governance Innovation, Waterloo.

Mian, A. and Sufi, A. (2014). *House of Debt: How They (and You) Caused the Great Recession, and How We Can Prevent It from Happening Again.* University of Chicago Press, Chicago.

Mian, A. and Sufi, A. (2018). "Finance and Business Cycles: The Credit-Driven Household Demand Channel," *Journal of Economic Perspectives,* 32(3), Summer, 31–58.

Mian, A., Sufi, A. and Verner, E. (2017). "Household Debt and Business Cycles Worldwide," *The Quarterly Journal of Economics,* 132(4), November, 1755–1817.

Milne, F. (2009). "The Complexities of Financial Risk Management and Systemic Risks," *Bank of Canada Review,* Summer, pp.15–29.

Office of the Superintendent of Financial Institutions (2020). "Liquidity Principles," January.

Rajan, R. G. (2005). "Has Financial Development Made the World Riskier?" NBER Working Paper No. 11728, November.

Schularick, M. and Taylor, A. M. (2012). "Credit Booms Gone Bust: Monetary Policy, Leverage Cycles, and Financial Crises, 1870–2008," *American Economic Review,* 102(2), April, 1029–1061.

Chapter 4

Plans and Preparations

1. Introduction

In Chapter 2, we described substantial weaknesses in the preparation by public health authorities and governments for the COVID-19 pandemic. These weaknesses increased the health and economic costs of the pandemic relative to what they would have been if preexisting recommendations had been followed and a wider set of plans had been put into place, including ones that would have better recognized the important interconnections between a pandemic, the overall effects on health of the population, and the economic consequences.

In this chapter, we set forth recommendations for carrying out postmortems on the COVID-19 experience, planning for future pandemics, and establishing a transparent and accountable governance regime for ongoing implementation of all the elements of a pre-pandemic plan. These three areas are important in and of themselves, as well as for setting the groundwork for the pandemic stress tests and exercise/wargames recommended in Chapter 5.

In Section 2 of this chapter, we explore pre-COVID reports and exercises (also known as wargames).[1] Many reports were not followed up or

---

[1] In Section 2.1, we provide a representative sample of exercises and reports. The WHO has a standard guide for country exercises and subsequent reports and recommendations. See https://apps.who.int/iris/bitstream/handle/10665/276175/WHO-WHE-CPI-2018.48-eng.pdf?sequence=1&isAllowed=y.

were poorly implemented. As well, some representative examples reveal the serious limitations in previous reports and exercises in that they were limited to the health consequences, the economic and social consequences of policies were ignored, and the report recommendations were often largely ignored. Furthermore, the pandemic models had major limitations that made it difficult to formulate policy. The problems with forecasting models are well known in many other areas. For example, we summarize the problems in finance models showing the limitations of predictive model methodology.

Section 3 of this chapter argues that the shortcomings in the current pandemic need to be identified in postmortems and taken into account in plans for future pre-pandemic and pandemic actions. We outline the key elements for postmortems. The postmortems and subsequent plans need to be shared across all levels of government (and governance) so that nothing falls between the cracks at the planning stage. A side benefit of this planning is that some of it will be useful for broader public health and economic readiness for other major catastrophes.

Drawing on Crean and Milne (2022), Section 4 outlines how a private catastrophe insurance scheme with a major government backstop would function to reduce banks' catastrophe risks and locate and manage those risks in a pre-packaged catastrophe insurance system.

Section 5 of the chapter takes a set of plans and institutions as given and argues for an appropriate governance system. It is not enough to have plans and recommendations coming out of exercises and wargames: It is too easy to have them written up and forgotten. They must be used to prepare for future emergencies. This requires a robust governance system that puts a high priority on transparency and accountability. Apart from the executive (or cabinet) branch of government, which will always play the key role, there should be three important elements of governance: semi-independent agencies to arrange for postmortems, propose pandemic plans, and implement some key elements of the approved plans; independent evaluation agencies to evaluate the implementation of the official pandemic plans, their updating, and the training of staff and those involved in governance regarding the plan and its importance; and the legislature and legislative committees that should review postmortems, plans, and reports of evaluation agencies. We discuss two examples of evaluation agencies.

The first is from the evaluation procedures of certain international organizations, as illustrated by those of the World Bank and the IMF. The second builds on existing roles of Auditors General (or Comptroller Generals). We outline their basic goals, procedures, and limitations.

In Section 6, we discuss some serious issues of organizational culture — inertia and obfuscation — and possible political corruption that can impede the governance system. We discuss bureaucratic and political impediments to effective planning and implementation, using a case study as an illustration. We argue that having a set of plans, which are transparent and for which institutions are accountable, along with a good governance system, should work to minimize these problems.

Section 7 concludes our discussion.

2. Pre-COVID-19 Pandemic Exercises and Reports

2.1 *A partial history of pandemic exercises and reports*

In the first year or so of the COVID-19 virus epidemic, the media discussed examples of previous epidemics, the public response, follow-up reports, and what was done in response. These reports and the lack of subsequent policy action were not encouraging.

2.1.1 *US forensic report on the 2014–2015 Ebola pandemic*

The Ebola epidemic was first diagnosed in West Africa in 2014. The World Health Organization (WHO) did not have the resources to respond adequately. The US, realizing this was potentially a very dangerous international pandemic, responded to seal off the virus before it spread and provided aid to West Africa. A number of lessons, summarized in a forensic report by Kirchhoff (2016), were learned from this episode.

The report discussed lessons that dealt with the lack of preparation in organizations, poor communication across agencies, the lack of appropriate equipment, and ineffective response strategies. Widespread international mobility made pandemic transmission an increasing risk. Kirchhoff observed that humanitarian, military, and health responders were not prepared when running periodic wargames.

Another important finding was the limited use of pandemic modeling in predicting outcomes and strategies. The standard models in use at that time proved seriously deficient in predicting the spread of the pandemic and incorporating social behavior and its impact into the propagation and severity of the virus.

In a recent interview, Kirchhoff (2020) observed that these deficiencies had not been rectified in the US.[2] The deficiencies had become apparent when COVID-19 hit the US.

2.1.2 *The US pandemic wargame in 2019*

In March 2020, the New York Times leaked a report of a 2019 wargame of a simulated "Crimson Contagion" in the US.[3] The report dealt almost exclusively with the health, organizational, and communication deficiencies that appeared in the game. This was an important wargame that found organizational and communication weaknesses in the Federal and State agencies that would deal with a pandemic.

Both the game and the Kirchhoff Report make no mention of the economic, financial, fiscal, and social implications of government strategies to contain the virus. If economists and other experts had been consulted, the economic, social, and fiscal consequences of various strategies should have been gamed and/or simulated. This chapter and Chapter 5 will explore this deficiency in detail.

Similar observations apply to many other countries. The US had at least made some preparations. Had other countries created forensic reports and/or acted on them?

2.1.3 *The 2006 Ontario SARS commission report*

Another example of public policy failure was an Ontario-commissioned 2006 report on the SARS outbreak in Ontario in the early 2000s.[4] The report was damning, arguing that the Ontario health system was

---

[2] See Kirchhoff (2020).
[3] See The New York Times (2020).
[4] See SARS Commission Report, Ontario (2006).

underfunded and woefully unprepared for a major epidemic. It made a number of recommendations to increase preparedness in equipment, organizations, and funding. In a Royal Society of Canada (2020) report, it has been alleged by experts in the area that these recommendations were ignored. Media reports have revealed disgraceful and tragic results in some Ontario nursing homes, where lack of preparation and public monitoring led to many deaths and suffering in squalid conditions.

2.1.4 *A history of national and international pandemic wargames*

The US and Ontario cases are not isolated examples: They are representative of a systemic problem. An April 2020 Canadian magazine article revealed a long history of national and international pandemic wargames beginning with the HIV outbreak in the 1980s.[5] The report summarized some of the games and responses. It is not clear if these games explored economic, financial, and fiscal implications of various quarantine strategies. But, it does quote several senior health and political figures involved in the games, saying that little had been done in many countries to use the games to influence policy and organizational structures; neither were the games used consistently to prepare senior policymakers for implementing the best policy responses in various plausible strategic scenarios.

2.2 *Pandemic computer models: Strengths and limitations*

As we discussed in detail in Chapter 2, computer models are one of the major tools used in constructing strategies combatting an epidemic. There is well-developed literature on computer simulation models of epidemics. A recent, detailed survey summarized different pre-COVID-19 methodologies in constructing predictive models of pandemics, exploring their strengths and limitations.[6]

---

[5] See Macleans, https://www.macleans.ca/news/world/the-doomed-30-year-battle-to-stop-a-pandemic/.

[6] See Chowell *et al.* (2016) and see also *The Economist* article reporting over- and underestimation of the severity of the epidemic. Many of these pre-Covid-19 models were updated to fit the recent data. https://www.economist.com/graphic-detail/2020/05/23/early-projections-of-covid-19-in-america-underestimated-its-severity.

Models help us organize our thoughts, use scientific and economic theories and information to explore effects and policies, and estimate or assign (based on history, theory, or experience) numerical parameters so we know which effects are large and which are small. Models can be helpful in assessing the outcomes of various policies. As well, they are useful for learning. Models can be compared to see which of them performed best as we observe outcomes. When models perform poorly, they lead researchers to try to find out the reasons why. When new data become available, models can be re-estimated or new variables or factors can be included. Indeed, in pandemic models, one would expect successive improvement as more data become available or when it becomes increasingly obvious which prediction biases from oversimplifications can be reduced by adding, in an appropriate way, a limited amount of additional complexity to the model.

Models have well-known strengths and limitations of which all modelers are, or should be, aware. As the famous statistician George Box observed, "All models are wrong but some are useful."[7] He elaborated on the evolution of models, their useful attributes, and their limitations:

> "One important idea is that science is a means whereby learning is achieved, not by mere theoretical speculation on the one hand, nor by the undirected accumulation of practical facts on the other, but rather by a motivated iteration between theory and practice ... The good scientist must have the flexibility and courage to seek out, recognize, and exploit such errors — especially his own. In particular, using Bacon's analogy, he must not be like Pygmalion and fall in love with his model...
>
> Since all models are wrong the scientist cannot obtain a "correct" one by excessive elaboration. On the contrary, following William of Occam, he should seek an economical description of natural phenomena. Just as the ability to devise simple but evocative models is the signature of the great scientist so overelaboration and over parameterization is often the mark of mediocrity.
>
> Since all models are wrong the scientist must be alert to what is importantly wrong. It is inappropriate to be concerned about mice when there are tigers abroad."[8]

---

[7] See Box (1976).
[8] *Ibid.*, pp. 791–792.

Creating a useable suite of predictive models is an iterative process. One can start with an abstract theory, formulated as equations relating the variables under study. (Usually, these theories have evolved from previous attempts to explain some phenomenon.) To make it operational, the model will have parameters to generate numerical outcomes. The parameters will be estimated from past data — and invariably estimated with error. Careful statisticians, econometricians, and modelers of all kinds will try various estimation methods and models to try to improve the estimation of key parameters, including, importantly, those on policy variables.

The next stage inserts the parameter estimates into the theoretical model and generates predictions for a future period. In a world that is evolving, there are various scenarios that could be anticipated, including those for various policies and various assumptions about human behavior and responses to policy. The model can be run under these scenarios to generate predictions conditional on each scenario. The final stage is to wait and observe what happened over the period that was predicted, and check the model's predictions with actual outcomes. (This part of the process is often referred to back-testing a model.)

As the model is an approximation, the modeler will look for systematic biased predictions and begin the iterative process of model improvement and testing again. Hopefully, the process converges to a useable set of models that will provide useful predictions for policy purposes. Unfortunately, much of the world is not so easily explained as it evolves physically and — in the case of human behavior — there are innovations that may have not been foreseen.

The pandemic class of models reflects the evolutionary process and difficulties that we have just discussed. They have a number of well-known strengths and limitations which modelers freely acknowledge:

1. Models are crucial for making policy decisions in the social sciences. For example, economists have long used models to help policymakers decide taxation policies, monetary policies, fiscal policies, and many other policy areas. Pandemic modeling is another area where decisions must be made about physical distancing, the use of masks, quarantine isolation, vaccination proportions in the population, etc. Without modeling and numerical estimation, political and health decisions would be based on very limited understanding of the impact of

various policy choices, and can lead to large, avoidable social, health, and economic costs.

2. Given data limitations, the evolution of the pandemic, etc., policy-makers are often faced with a suite of models that appear to approximately fit the data, but have significant differences in policy implications. As the pandemic evolves, new data are collected and there are revisions of the models, and policies will adjust to the new analysis. But, when major differences in model predictions persist, they create serious policy problems. When different models consistently give very different results, that have major consequences for policy decisions, the authorities are faced with a quandary. Competent, honest modelers will try to find the causes for the differing predictions. Here are some possible areas that should be explored:

   (a) Data may not be available, at least initially, on key variables or factors. Modelers may have based parameter estimates on different proxy variables or tried other modeling devices to address the issue.

   (b) The different models may use different theoretical structures, some simple, some complex. These modeling choices are unavoidable. As Box observed, complexity does not guarantee added predictive power. For example, a complex model may defy the modeler's intuition, so that, in some cases, predictions may be significantly affected by coding errors that are subtle and difficult to detect.

   (c) Model results provide a range of outcomes *conditional* on different estimated social/health policies. Pandemic models predict time profiles of infection and mortality rates *conditional* on the parameters, the human responses through time to policy, and the policies undertaken. Unconditional predictions provide poor predictions and can be highly misleading beyond the first few weeks.

   (d) Back-testing reveals the limitations of some of these predictive models.[9]

---

[9] A recent study by Funk *et al.* (2019) used the Ebola virus outbreak in 2013–16 to test the reliability of standard models. This study showed reliable predictions out to one or two weeks, but there was increasing unreliability for longer periods, reflecting the high degree of uncertainty in the processes driving the models: https://journals.plos.org/ploscompbiol/article/file?id=10.1371/journal.pcbi.1006785&type=printable.

The limitations of pandemic models are not restricted to this class of predictive models, but are common in almost all other areas of science and economics where predictive models are used.[10] We will give an example to illustrate the limitations of predictive models.

2.2.1 *Example 1: Financial risk management models*

Risk managers and financial regulators have long grappled with the limitations of modeling financial markets, credit, market funding, liquidity, and systemic risks.[11] The fundamental issues that we saw in pandemic models have been recognized in financial risk management models: data limitations, model choices, strategic choices impacting outcomes, etc.

Model back-testing is standard practice in attempting to validate financial models. Many models show their limitations in back-tests, especially in Plausible Worst Case (PWC) events. PWC events are extremely difficult to predict with statistical models because extreme data points are sparse and/or non-stationary, and model predictions often lack statistical and predictive robustness.

Some statistical models attempt to accommodate PWC events by modeling distributions with "fat tails." But, these models rely on very few data points in the tail, so that distribution parameters are estimated with a serious lack of precision.

To complement the statistical models used for "normal" times, financial stress tests are widely used to deal with PWC tail events. In some limited cases, financial wargames are used for PWC downside scenarios. We will explore these techniques in more detail in Chapter 5.

See also the paper by Ioannidis, Cripps, and Tanner (2020) which is highly critical of many forecasting models used in the COVID crisis.

[10] See the excellent discussion by a mathematician, economist, and climate scientist: https://www.youtube.com/watch?time_continue=1&v=5MoE1-Fi-Ko&feature= emb_logo.

[11] See the text book discussion of market risk modeling by Dowd (2005), *Measuring Market Risk*, Second Edition, Wiley 2005. See also Milne (2009) for detailed discussions of the problems with risk management models, particularly credit, liquidity, and systemic risks since the financial crisis of 2007–2009. https://www.bankofcanada.ca/wp-content/ uploads/2010/06/milne1.pdf.

We turn now to the current pandemic and discuss the essential elements for creating an effective postmortem.

3. Postmortems and Plans

3.1 *Postmortems as the pandemic is coming to an end*

Postmortems were essential following the GFC to improve financial regulation. Similarly, they will be important to improve future pandemic planning.

Typically, there would have been plans by regional/local health authorities, provincial/state authorities, and national authorities for pandemics. These plans would typically have had two components: preparation prior to the pandemic and strategies employed during the pandemic. It is important that at each of the three governmental levels postmortems be carried out to see whether preparation plans prior to the pandemic had been carried out, what other plans for preparations should have been made, whether the advance plans for actions during a pandemic had been carried out in a timely manner (and if not why), and what was learned that should be included in any future pandemic planning.

Those writing the postmortems need to have independence so that their views are not tarnished by those who failed to take effective action before or during the pandemic. Although the postmortems at the three levels of governance (national, provincial/state/regional, local/small regions) should be largely conducted independently, there need to be consultations across levels on issues that are the responsibility of more than one level. Importantly, a process needs to be put in place so that misunderstandings and miscommunication across these levels both before and during the pandemic can be recognized in these reports. The purpose of these postmortems is to improve the situation for the next pandemic, not to assign blame. All these postmortems need to be specific about their recommendations, transparent about shortcomings, and made publicly available.

Depending on which level of governance is being considered, these postmortems in the area of public health will need to deal with such topics as the presence, implementation, appropriateness, and effectiveness of the following:

- Past plans for sufficient availability of personal protective equipment (in the health care sector writ large, long-term care homes, and for employees in other sectors), ventilators, other equipment, health care workers and personal support workers, and hospital space.
- Past conventions for updating plans, making them transparent, and ensuring that they are being followed before a pandemic.
- Past clarity in federations or countries with regional health authorities of the role of the national government in providing additional personal protective equipment, ventilators, and other equipment.
- Past plans (or options) regarding the closure of national or provincial/state borders to movement of people.
- Past plans to deal with identified operational risks such as health care and personal support workers being employed at more than one site, and laboratory capacity to process tests for a disease.
- Past plans to ramp up testing and contact tracing capabilities quickly.
- Past plans to collect comprehensive, comparable data on cases and deaths from a pandemic disease in a manner that is easily shared and aggregated.
- Past plans to collect and quickly disseminate comparable data on all deaths by cause in a manner that is easily shared and aggregated.
- Past plans taking into account the possible effects of public health restrictions on mental health and the health of those whose surgeries may be put off indefinitely.
- Past plans giving guidance on the clarity of messages to the public.
- Past plans considering the spread of communicable diseases in particular workplaces where workers work very closely with one another and in particular residences, such as long-term care homes, prisons, and migrant worker dormitories.
- Past plans for the possible use of masks and their supply to the general public.

Public health postmortems will also have to identify other areas where there was insufficient planning before the pandemic, as well as where insufficient planning and decision-making were undertaken between the first and second (and further subsequent) waves. The way that evidence from other countries was taken into account during the pandemic in planning and decision-making should also be examined.

Importantly, new lessons from this pandemic about planning for future pandemics need to be noted.

Expertise in pandemic-related areas (especially with hands-on experience) should be the key requirement for inclusion in teams performing the postmortems. The teams should exclude senior officials who were responsible for much of the implementation of preexisting plans, but could (and often should) include former senior officials. They should include at least one senior person from outside the jurisdiction and (at the national and provincial/state level) at least one other senior person from another institution within the jurisdiction.

The postmortem teams should consult with those in the relevant fields who are known to think outside the box, including, importantly, those who made significant contributions to knowledge, interpretation, and practices over the course of the pandemic. As well, outside-the-box thinkers whose ideas were ignored, but later appreciated, need to be consulted.[12]

In addition to postmortems in the public health area, provincial/state and national governments need to conduct postmortems on what information and public policy preparation were missing, and what needs to go into planning for the next pandemic. Information would include the following: the input/output relationships among industries that could affect the transmission of lockdowns; the special surveys that should be commissioned from national statistical agencies and private polling companies during a pandemic; and the methods for dealing with transfer of payments (including unemployment insurance), loans to firms and individuals, and subsidies to firms. Financial regulators should conduct postmortems (both nationally and internationally) on the appropriateness and effectiveness of various temporary changes in regulation or guidance during the pandemic — including those regarding foreclosures and delays in loan repayments.

---

[12] Lewis (2021) covers the stories of a number of Americans whose outside-the-box thinking made important contributions to dealing with the Covid-19 pandemic in the United States.

All postmortems need to be thorough, transparent, and made publicly available. Provincial/state and national postmortems should be discussed in legislative committees and legislatures.

Learning from mistakes and unpreparedness in this pandemic is one of the major ways to prepare for the future. However, it must be recognized that no two pandemics will be the same.

3.2 *Planning for future pandemics*

Postmortems are really only valuable to the extent that they lead to better planning and implementation in the future, both in the area of public health and the area of economic and social policy.

It is clear that much has already been learned from the experience of the current pandemic, from the evident gaps noted by many, including public health professionals themselves and journalists (recall our Chapter 2). Some postmortems have already begun, as in the three focused ones by the Auditor-General of Ontario (2020), discussed in more detail in the next section.

Public health planning for future pandemics will, by its very nature, have two components: pre-pandemic planning and plans for actions that will need to take place during a pandemic itself.

Pre-pandemic planning will need to include but not be restricted to the following:

- Keeping an up-to-date stock of personal protective equipment, ventilators, and other equipment, extra hospital space, and laboratory capacity.
- Ensuring rapid productive capacity or securing supply chains for mRNA or other effective vaccines for the particular virus.[13]

---

[13] mRNA vaccines have been developed to provide rapid responses to new virus strains. See https://www.nature.com/articles/nrd.2017.243 and https://www.uab.edu/news/youcanuse/item/12059-covid-19-mrna-vaccines-how-could-anything-developed-this-quickly-be-safe.

- Putting into place and testing data systems which will allow data to be collected, rapidly disseminated, and shared in an analytic-friendly and research-friendly manner.
- Establishing and implementing standards for the design of long-term care facilities, seniors' homes, migrant worker housing, and housing for the currently homeless, and ensuring that are sufficient such facilities.
- Providing adequate training regarding pandemic procedures and personal protective equipment for personal care workers and certain other health care workers.
- Establishing norms for the extent to which personal care workers, nurses, and other health professionals can work in more than one location over the course of the week.

Planning needs to take into account that pandemics can be of varying intensities. It must contemplate pandemics that are much worse than those that have been observed this time around.

Plans for what is to be done in the public health domain during pandemics themselves will have to include most of the other specific areas set out in the discussion of postmortems earlier in this chapter.

Plans in the economic policy action area will consist of gathering necessary economic data both prior to and during the pandemic, and setting out and evaluating policy options — including transfers to individuals, wage subsidies, other subsidies to firms, and loans to firms — that could be used in a pandemic. Any policy option that is evaluated as being a highly appropriate option should then lead to the construction of computer and other systems necessary to support and implement the strategy. The supporting logistics are critical for effective implementation.

Plans for monetary and fiscal policy need to be conditional on the distance from the effective lower bound on interest rates and the preexisting real yields on government debt.

All pandemic plans need to be shared across levels of governance so that nothing falls between the cracks at the planning stage. It is important to note that a side benefit of this planning is that some of it will be useful for broader public health and economic preparation for other major environmental or strategic shocks and policy actions. As one example, proponents of an extension of "basic income" have noted the need for appropriate computer and other systems to implement such a policy.

3.3 *Cost–benefit and studies of policy options*

The COVID pandemic has provided a rich set of policy problems. At the beginning of the pandemic, there was a great deal of uncertainty about the degree of contagion and lethality of the virus. Many governments instituted strict rules on social distancing, requiring citizens to wear masks and introducing quarantines and border controls of varying degrees of severity. Each of these policies has benefits and costs. Relying on early modeling predictions, many policymakers judged that strict measures reduced the rate of infection and allowed the medical system to treat seriously ill patients without being overwhelmed. The costs of these policies in terms of business shutdowns, delayed surgeries, etc., were judged to be manageable given various polices introduced to ameliorate the negative consequences of lockdowns. Within the first few months, it became clear that the elderly and those with comorbidities were the segment of the population most at risk. Long-term care homes had been hard hit by the virus, leading to a high proportion of deaths.

Subsequently, modified policies were introduced for patients in long-term care homes and more targeted restrictions to safeguard the most vulnerable. These policies have continued to evolve, as new vaccines were produced earlier than many expected, and new and more virulent strains of the virus appeared leading to subsequent waves of infections and deaths.

When choosing among the policy options for this pandemic, there is a sequence of decisions that must be made given the information at any time. This is a difficult iterative process as revised information appears.[14] At any time, the following should occur:

(a) Policymakers must understand the current information about the virus, particularly the demographics of those at risk and the effectiveness of various treatments.
(b) They should understand the capacity of their health system in response to varying degrees of severity of the pandemic.
(c) They should use a suite of models to try to understand the impact on the virulence and lethality of the virus given any set of policy choices.

---

[14] For an insightful discussion, see Carney (2021) Chapters 9 and 10.

(d) There should be models that give predictions of the economic, social, and health costs of policies that are a consequence of the policies used to combat the virus.

(e) They should attempt to estimate the dynamics of policy choices, understanding that policies will have short-term and long-term consequences.

(f) Given the possible outcomes, policymakers will have the difficult ethical task of choosing over vectors of feasible outcomes.

(g) Members of society may well disagree over policy choices given their interpretation of evidence, model choices, and ethical weights over outcomes.[15]

(h) Given the evolution of information, the policy process will iterate through the previous steps. Over time, policy changes may just reflect this sensible iterative process.[16]

There have been various attempts to calculate the benefits and costs of various policies to combat the pandemic. In the early stages of the pandemic, strong quarantine restrictions (lockdowns of varying degrees) reduced the spread and severity of the virus — this benefit was very apparent. But, as the pandemic evolved, the policy options became more nuanced given the effectiveness of the new vaccines.

We turn now to the costs of various quarantine restrictions and strong lockdowns. Policymakers must estimate the following:

(a) The economic costs of lockdowns in lost production and disruption.

(b) The major income and wealth redistributions consequences of shutting down non-essential industries. Many professional workers were able to work online and suffered mere inconvenience. Firms that provided services on the Internet saw demand increase, leading to

---

[15] See Carney (2021) Chapter 10 for the difficulties in computing costs and benefits, given the uncertainty over outcomes. Also, there are various ways of measuring the value of a life for different age groups. Any precise numerical answer to these calculations provides spurious precision to a complex set of problems.

[16] This process requires a careful and transparent communication policy so that media commentators are not tempted to use 20–20 hindsight to unfairly criticize sensible policy evolution.

increased profits and stock prices.[17] Conversely, workers in hospitality and other inessential industries lost their jobs, and many small businesses went bankrupt. Although there were fiscal subsidy and loan schemes, their efficiency and effectiveness have been patchy. The impact of lockdown policies on the poor in the Global South is deeply worrying.[18]

(c) The sharp policy focus on the virus has reduced the diagnosis, treatment, and surgery for heart, cancer, and other major medical conditions.[19] This has major implications for future health outcomes.

(d) In many jurisdictions, schools and tertiary education institutions abandoned face-to-face instruction, replacing it with online teaching. There have been numerous complaints that this has disadvantaged poor children who have limited online facilities and family help. Many students complain that online courses are an inferior substitute for face-to-face teaching. This is especially true for elementary and secondary school students.

It is too early to make a definitive analysis of various policies to combat the virus, because the pandemic is continuing, and the costs and benefits are evolving. For example, Helliwell, Norton, Wang, and Wang (2021) have conducted a well-being analysis across countries. They concluded that the elimination strategy followed by Japan, South Korea, Australia, New Zealand, and Iceland was superior to less stringent strategies followed by other Western countries. The study was based on 2020 data. A danger with elimination strategies in isolated societies, however, is that the population will see no urgency in vaccination. When the virus does spread, then the country is faced with rising infections and a lightly vaccinated population.[20] Thus, the results in mid-2021 in some of the countries that did follow an elimination strategy, such as Australia and

---

[17] Amazon is a well-known example.

[18] For an analysis, see Green (2021).

[19] For example, see the UK National Health service under stress: https://www.bmj.com/content/bmj/372/bmj.n215.full.pdf and https://www.bhf.org.uk/what-we-do/news-from-the-bhf/news-archive/2021/may/lives-at-risk-from-ticking-timebomb-in-cardiovascular-care-warns-charity.

[20] By August 2021 some states in Australia were facing rapidly rising infection rates.

Japan, were not as positive as in 2020. COVID cases and deaths rose, and so did non-COVID health, social, and economic costs.

In a survey of cost–benefit studies, Allen [21] summarized and evaluated 80 studies of the impact of COVID policies. He found that many studies overestimated the benefits of strong lockdown policies and underestimated the costs. He re-estimated the cost–benefit ratio for Canada and concluded, "…it is possible that lockdown will go down as one of the greatest peacetime policy failures in Canada's history." This conclusion, however, is subject to many assumptions, including the relative response of output (GDP) to deaths, cases, and lockdowns over both the near term and the longer term.

Indeed, ex-post evaluation of policies is a very contentious issue that requires further serious study. For example, as the pandemic has evolved, vaccinations have become a feasible policy tool. In mid-2020, most policymakers appeared to assume that workable vaccines would not appear until mid or late 2021. Hindsight should not be used to criticize policies that were implemented in the first half of 2020, given the knowledge available at the time.

Current knowledge surrounding the effectiveness of the available vaccines is evolving. Current vaccines may or may not be as effective against new mutations. As the information about vaccines evolves, policies will change to account for their effectiveness, and the likelihood of the introduction of modified and improved vaccines.

Careful policy and implementation planning for a future pandemic should summarize the lessons of previous pandemics (including the COVID episode) understanding the cost–benefit consequences of various health, economic, and social responses.

4. Catastrophe Risk Insurance[22]

This section examines the reaction of the financial system to the COVID-19 crisis. During 2020, uncertainties about the ultimate scale of

---

[21] See Douglas W. Allen "Covid Lockdown Cost/Benefits" A Critical Assessment of the Literature" (2021), https://www.sfu.ca/~allen/LockdownReport.pdf.

[22] This section is a very brief summary of a far more detailed study. See Crean and Milne (2022).

bank loan losses stemming from COVID-19 led to bank equity capital conservation measures, including tightened lending standards that impeded bank lending to financially stretched customers. The section identifies three major areas of national unpreparedness that led to this result. First, the Basel III-compliant risk management processes of banks are not structured to identify catastrophic risk, leaving material, unrecognized catastrophe risk in bank portfolios with no layer of capital to absorb such risk. Second, the insurance industry, which uses risk techniques designed to identify catastrophic risk, does not have the capacity for providing adequate property and casualty coverage for catastrophes. Third, most western governments have failed to develop detailed preparations to contain the impact of potential catastrophes and to assist individuals and firms to recover in the wake of a catastrophe.

Following the outbreak of COVID-19, most governments mounted expedited programs of direct governmental financial assistance to firms and individuals. However, since governments lack proper data on proposed recipients, and they lack the systems and trained personnel to evaluate the data, the programs resulted in substantial wastage. Assistance was provided to some firms and individuals that had sufficient funding of their own. Inadequate assistance was provided to firms which, with proper support, would have remained viable and their employment saved. The losses of many small and medium firms can be attributed to such shortcomings. And, assistance was provided to firms which had no business potential for viability.

Crean and Milne (2022) argue that the most effective solution to these nested problems begins by tackling the insurance protection gaps, particularly the property and business interruption coverage gaps. This should be done through legislated government backstops on the model of the existing terrorism and nuclear accident insurance. With appropriate backstops, the market growth in catastrophe coverage would largely close the protection gaps. Insurance policies then would cover the losses of firms caused by the catastrophe and would largely replace the heavy charges to the equity base of firms from catastrophe losses and thereby protect the viability of such firms. Such claims proceeds would substantially reduce the extent of direct government support needed in the absence of adequate insurance coverage. Since insurance companies have the appropriate data, systems, and personnel to administer such policies, the claims payouts will be delivered in a much more highly targeted fashion than the assistance provided under government-administered programs.

In addition, personal insurance for employees could be added to unemployment insurance for employees of marginal firms that cannot survive lockdowns. One component of the firm insurance would be to provide incentives for firms to retain employees who otherwise would have been lost, thus destroying valuable firm-specific human capital.

Closing catastrophe coverage gaps will largely remove catastrophe risks from bank portfolios. Catastrophes should no longer cause surges in bank loan losses. Bank lending standards should not behave pro-cyclically after a catastrophe, and bank customers will have access to normal availability of new loans. This can replace much of the need for government-administered loan programs and will do so in a much more targeted and efficient fashion.

5. Governance, Evaluation, and Accountability for Planning and Preparedness

5.1 *Introduction*

It is not enough to have postmortems and plans (and stress tests and exercises): It is too easy for these to be written up and ignored. The reports must be used in preparing for future emergencies. This requires a robust governance system that puts a high priority on transparency, accountability, and enforcement of the plans and recommendations. This is true whether one is considering international organizations, national governments, provincial/state/regional governments, or local or regional public health authorities.

Mark Carney, among others, has noted three behavioral reasons why governments may not be well prepared for disasters of various kinds, including pandemics.[23] The first is recency bias, whereby more importance is given to recent events rather than historical ones. The second is disaster myopia, whereby the probability of adverse outcomes is underestimated, as often seems to be the case for low-frequency high-cost events such as disasters. The third is hyperbolic discounting, a time-inconsistent

---

[23] Carney (2021).

model of discounting the future in which the value that individuals or institutions ascribe to future payoffs falls rapidly after the near term.[24] Hyperbolic discounting arises from having a "present bias." With such discounting, government expenditures with definite payoffs this year may be preferred to expenditures on training for pandemics or health infrastructure that would have the payoff in the future of lowering the cost of a pandemic. It is important to note that all three of these behavioral reasons are likely to be at play among large parts of the electorate, the bureaucracy, and the politicians who ultimately make decisions on whether plans will be followed and expenditures made.

Given these behaviors, which are "irrational" in the sense that, ex ante, the vast majority of people would argue that it is important that countries pay to be well prepared for pandemics, we seek to find governance models that would minimize the chance of irrational, time-inconsistent behavior of governments and their agencies.

Paul Tucker has written on the problem of governments being able to credibly commit to stick to an agreed-upon policy or plan, and whether an agency with a degree of independence would be able to stick to the policy or plan while having the legitimacy to be able to continue to play the role as its implementer.[25]

In democracies, we see there being four areas where there is a potential role for an agency or agencies with at least some degree of independence so as to give unbiased views and/or make credible commitments:

- Carrying out postmortems and putting together plans for pandemic preparation
- Implementing (parts of) the plan not involving capital expenditures
- Designing and reporting on stress tests and exercises
- Evaluating whether the plan has been put into place and is being updated regularly.

The first three of these roles could potentially be played by a pandemic planning section hived off from a public health agency. We consider this in some detail in the next section.

---

[24] This differs from normal exponential discounting.
[25] Tucker (2018).

The last role would more likely be played by an Auditor General (or Comptroller General),[26] or by the type of independent evaluation office used in international organizations such as the World Bank or International Monetary Fund. We consider this role in more detail in Section 5.3.

In considering the governance of the pandemic planning process overall, it is also important to consider the role of the legislature in establishing a governance and review system, and the role of legislative committees in reviewing postmortem reports, plans, reports on stress tests and pandemics, and reports evaluating progress with respect to putting the plan into place. We come back to this in Section 5.4.

Although all these issues are relevant to the international level and local public health authorities as well, they are particularly important at the national and province/state/region level. Therefore, our specific analysis in Sections 5.2 through 5.4 focuses on those two levels, including their legislatures. Some of the analysis would apply in a general way to the international and local public health authorities as well, but we do not consider the details (except in the case of evaluation agencies in international organizations).

5.2 *An agency for planning, updating the plan, testing the plan, and maybe more*

Many public health agencies are, among other things, responsible for infectious diseases and emergency preparedness and response. Thus, they are already responsible for having an emergency plan for a pandemic, for updating the plan, and (in principle) testing out the plan as well. In addition, they would be responsible for implementing any parts of the plan for preparations that are intended to be carried out directly by the public health agency itself, as opposed to by other parts of the government more involved, for example, with hospitals and long-term care facilities (or procurement or storage of stockpiles of equipment).

---

[26] In Australia, the post is known as the Auditor-General (in the Australian National Audit Office); in Canada, the Auditor General; in the United Kingdom, the Comptroller and Auditor General (in the National Audit Office); and in the United States, the Comptroller General (in the Government Accountability Office).

For the reasons of recency bias, disaster myopia, hyperbolic discounting, and the credible commitment problem, it would be useful for there to be an agency with independence to carry out the planning, updating, testing, and implementation of the preparations plan.

However, it does not seem that this could be a fully "independent agency" as defined by Paul Tucker, with job-secure policymakers, control over policy instruments, and "some autonomy in determining" its budget.[27] Although job security could be granted, and an agency could be given control over putting together its preparation plans, it would not seem legitimate to have it actually implement those preparation plans for expenses to be made by other agencies, departments, or institutions, nor to implement some parts of those plans itself during an actual pandemic. As well, it is not clear how the agency could be given a fair degree of budgetary control, as needs could change considerably from decade to decade and the relative needs for direct spending by the agency and plan-related spending by other institutions could vary considerably through time.

Nonetheless, having an agency with some degree of independence to deal with pandemic planning, updating, and testing would be very attractive. Tucker talks about information agencies, "independent bodies that produce information and give independent advice on policy." One could envisage a largely independent "information and pandemic planning" agency formed from the key sections within a public health agency dealing with emergency preparedness and response, as well as infectious diseases. It could either operate as a stand-alone agency, governed by its own statute, or as an agency within the public health agency, but mandated by the statute for the public health agency. The head of this new agency should be appointed for a long term of seven to ten years. As well, the statute creating the agency should be very specific about its planning responsibilities, including the updating and testing of plans. To identify this agency as one that is separate from the evaluation agency discussed in the next section, we will refer to it as the "pandemic planning agency."

---

[27] Paul Tucker, *op. cit.*

It would be important for the head of the agency and other senior employees to welcome outside-the-box thinking from within and outside the agency, especially when plans are updated.

Although this agency should largely cover health matters, it should also be responsible for the coordination for the testing of plans (stress tests and exercises) for associated fiscal matters.

5.3 *An agency to evaluate whether the plan is being put into place and is being updated*

The full extent of an evaluation role should include evaluating the following:

- The implementation of the official plan: Are pre-pandemic actions on track and specified targets being met? What is the overall state of readiness?
- Has the official plan incorporated recommendations from postmortems, exercises, and wargames?
- As required by an agreed-upon updating schedule, has the official plan been updated to incorporate new scientific/medical findings and new technologies?
- Are all senior staff and key personnel being trained in the content of relevant parts of the official plan and its importance?
- Are those in key governance roles (e.g., ministers) being trained regarding the key elements and importance of the plan?

In this section, we look at two possible models for agencies for evaluation. The first is a separate independent agency associated with a specific area. Examples here are from the World Bank and the International Monetary Fund. The second is from a traditional Auditor General (or Comptroller General) role.

For the World Bank, we outline their basic goals and procedures. Their oversight system provides a good guide of the issues that we wish to explore here.

The IMF has implemented a review system of their Evaluation process. The IMF review is important for it reveals how the results of evaluations (exercises or wargames) can be ignored, and not acted upon as a matter of course. This is very revealing in explaining bureaucratic impediments to action.

5.3.1 *The World Bank evaluation process*

The World Bank has set out the basic principles of its evaluation process as follows:

"In line with international practices in evaluation, evaluations in the World Bank Group system should adhere to three core principles that can help ensure the quality and effectiveness of evaluation.

1. **Utility**. Evaluation utility refers to the relevance and timeliness of evaluation processes and findings to organizational learning, decision making, and accountability for results.
2. **Credibility**: Without careful monitoring, important data cannot be collected. The availability of good monitoring data is necessary for good evaluation.
3. **Evaluation independence** is in place when the evaluation process is free from undue political influence and organizational pressure. Independence can be achieved through various mechanisms. Structural independence is ensured when the evaluation function has its own budget, staffing, and work plan that are not subject to approval by World Bank Group Management but directly under the supervision of the Board of Executive Directors for each institution (hereafter referred to as the "Boards"). Functional independence refers to the ability of the unit managing the evaluation to decide on what to evaluate and how to go about the evaluation. Finally, behavioral independence implies professional integrity and absence of bias in the attitude and behavioral conduct of the evaluator."[28]

---

[28] See the World Bank document for a full discussion: https://ieg.worldbankgroup.org/sites/default/files/Data/reports/WorldBankEvaluationPrinciples.pdf.

5.3.2 *The IMF's review of its evaluation process*[29]

The IMF created an Independent Evaluation Office (IEO) that has been in operation for many years.[30] The IEOs' purpose is summarized in the following paragraph:

"The Independent Evaluation Office (IEO) has been established to systematically conduct objective and independent evaluations on issues, and on the basis of criteria, of relevance to the mandate of the Fund. It is intended to serve as a means to enhance the learning culture within the Fund, strengthen the Fund's external credibility, and support the Executive Board's institutional governance and oversight responsibilities. IEO has been designed to complement the review and evaluation work within the Fund and should, therefore, improve the institution's ability to draw lessons from its experience and more quickly integrate improvements into its future work."

The IEO's purpose is similar to the World Bank's evaluation process — and that of many evaluation bodies attached to large private and public organizations. Although the details may vary across organizations, we will concentrate on the effectiveness of this type of review body in improving the operations of the main organization.

What is novel is that the IMF has been running periodic reviews of the IEO and its impact on the operations of the IMF. The findings of the Panel are summarized below[31]:

The IEO has too little impact in the Fund:
The Panel found that although the Board revealed goodwill toward the IEO, it had not been used effectively by the Board as an oversight and governance tool.

---

[29] This section draws upon the 2018 IMF document "Time for a reboot at a critical time for multilateralism: The Third External Evaluation of the IEO".
https://www.imf.org/en/News/Articles/2018/07/17/pr18296imf-executive-board-considers-external-evaluation-of-the-independent-evaluation-office.

[30] For the IEO's terms of reference, see https://ieo.imf.org/en/our-mandate/Terms-of-Reference.

[31] See the Executive Summary and the full document for details: https://www.imf.org/en/News/Articles/2018/07/17/pr18296imf-executive-board-considers-external-evaluation-of-the-independent-evaluation-office.

The context the IEO operates in has changed:
The IMF has changed; it has become much more transparent, and it is easier for the outside world to scrutinize its work. It has also demonstrated an ability to learn from its experiences and made significant changes to its surveillance and lending toolkit following the Global Financial Crisis. But increased public accountability and scrutiny imply that the IEO needs to be more vigilant and integrated into the management of the IMF.

The IEO risks becoming "routinized and bureaucratized":
A survey conducted of IMF staff reveals low awareness of the IEO's work, and interviews with senior staff generally report little learning value or relevance in IEO reports (with some exceptions). Learning was not embedded into the organization. Change was only at the level of measured activity — and showed substantial delays in implementation.

The root causes of the lack of traction were three-fold:

The Board has not consistently demonstrated to management and the IEO the importance it attaches to independent evaluation.

Management has not instilled the importance and value of the IEO's work in the IMF's senior staff, nor given incentives to shape desired behavior.

The IEO has not engaged sufficiently with management and staff at each stage of the evaluation to ensure understanding of each other's viewpoints so that the learning value of the evaluation can be maximized.

Although this critique deals specifically with the operations of the IEO, the failures are common to many review systems in large organizations. The lessons we can draw from this report are similar in substance to the lack of serious responses to pandemic wargames that we explored in Chapter 2. There were no serious reforms when these exercises revealed major deficiencies. Nor were there major adverse consequences for bureaucratic and political leadership when they failed to implement reforms. The review process fails if the lessons are not learned and acted upon. As we have observed in the COVID pandemic, the health, economic, and social costs are very high when there is a lack of adequate preparation.

5.3.3 *COVID-19 public policy case study: The Ontario Auditor General's report*[32]

As noted above, as opposed to having a specialized evaluation agency, one could rely on an existing Auditor General or Comptroller General to do evaluations.

In this section, we provide a case study of what an existing Auditor General has produced on certain issues related to the COVID-19 pandemic.

In November 2020, the Ontario Auditor General (OAG) reported on the province's response to the COVID-19 pandemic, its planning, the effectiveness of its case management, and contact tracing. The reports make lamentable reading. We provide a brief summary of their findings, paraphrased from the OAG news release.[33]

There had been significant changeover in leadership in Ontario's Provincial Emergency Management Office (EMO), outdated emergency plans and the lack of sufficient staff.

The Central Co-ordination Table held its first meeting almost a month into the emergency, on April 11, 2020. In contrast to Ontario, other provinces activated their existing response structures and emergency plans.

Key lessons identified in the aftermath of the Severe Acute Respiratory Syndrome (SARS) outbreak in 2003 had not been implemented by the time COVID-19 hit Ontario and were not followed during Ontario's COVID-19 response. The Auditors saw delays and confusion in decision-making.

The Chief Medical Officer of Health did not fully exercise his powers under the Health Protection and Promotion Act to respond to COVID-19.

Public Health Ontario played a diminished role in the overall provincial response, and even regional response structures were generally

---

[32] These reports can be accessed at: https://www.auditor.on.ca/en/content/news/news. html#2020.

[33] https://www.auditor.on.ca/en/content/news/specials_newsreleases/newsrelease_ COVID-19.pdf.

not led by public health experts. Local Medical Officers of Health informed the Auditor that they were confused by provincial politicians delivering critical public health advice in place of the Chief Medical Officer of Health.

Variations in management and operations among public health units contributed to fragmentation and inconsistencies across Ontario. Public health in other jurisdictions, such as British Columbia, Alberta and Quebec, is more simply organized. As of the writing of the report, Ontario's 34 public health units were still operating independently, and best practices were still often not being shared.

The Ministry of the Solicitor General did not implement recommendations made three years earlier to regularly update and finalize its emergency response plans. As well, the Ministry of Health had not acted on recommendations in the 2003, 2007, 2014, and 2017 audits to address the weaknesses in public health lab and information systems. This had negatively impacted the work of public health units during COVID-19. Information systems in use had limited functionality for case management and contact tracing. Also, the Ministry of Health did not make the improvements needed in its fragmented management of the laboratory sector. Laboratory testing still followed a substantially manual, paper-based process, and the laboratory information system was not integrated with the public health information system.

Ontario did not contact all travellers entering the province due to a lack of dedicated resources and the inability to receive accurate, complete and timely information from the federal government. Between April and August 2020, about 2.5 million international travellers entered Ontario. Approximately 9%, or 233,000, of them were reported to the Ontario authorities.

These failings were not uncommon in other provinces, states, or countries. There are some jurisdictions that have performed much better in being prepared, moving swiftly to implement policy actions that carefully balanced health, social, and economic factors. Nevertheless, the OAG report demonstrates that even when lessons were documented and reforms recommended, Ontario governments had ignored the recommendations made in the OAG's 2003, 2007, 2014, and 2017 audits.

5.3.4 *Summary on an agency to evaluate*

The evaluation role could be played well by either a stand-alone agency (as in the World Bank or IMF) or an Auditor General. Auditors General and their agency usually have independence: The Auditors General are typically officers of the legislature (not the executive), they are given long terms of office, and they have much independence in determining what to examine (and how to examine it) and much independence in allocating their budget. It would be important that a stand-alone evaluation agency for pandemic preparation have similar guarantees of independence. It would be important that the head of a stand-alone evaluation agency be in their final job within government so that they would be immune from hints of preferment.[34]

As the time since a pandemic occurred lengthens, it might seem that there is little for a stand-alone agency to do. This might favor an Auditor General playing the role. In that case, it would likely be important to have some permanent staff in the pandemic area to provide some continuity.

Whether the evaluation role is played by a stand-alone agency or the Auditor General, it would be important for legislation to clearly spell out the evaluation role in pandemic planning that is to be played.

5.4 *Role of the legislature and legislative committees*

The law establishing a new stand-alone agency or giving the Auditor General a very specific role in evaluating pandemic planning needs to have some specific clauses in it:

(a) Defining what is to be evaluated and requiring a list of recommendations to be made.
(b) Defining with what frequency it is to be evaluated.
(c) Allowing the government to see the report before it is made public so that its written response (indicating agreement or not with the recommendations) can be made at the same time as publication.
(d) Guaranteeing the publication of the report when it is tabled in the legislature.

---

[34] In private correspondence, Paul Tucker made a similar point to the authors.

(e) Stating that the report is to be sent to the legislative committee responsible for health (as well as the committee, such as the public accounts committee, that may receive all the other reports of an Auditor General).

(f) Requiring follow-up reports from the agency, within a specified period of time, on whether the government has implemented the recommendations it agreed with.

The role of the legislative committees in examining the reports of the evaluation agency and the reports and major plans of the pandemic planning agency is extremely important. It ensures the accountability of both the pandemic planning agency and the government in pandemic planning, as well as strongly encouraging the agency and government to have the will to act.[35] It would be important for the legislative committees to place emphasis on weaknesses in pandemic planning and for the media to stress the importance of dealing with these weaknesses. Presumably the legislative committee responsible for health would take the lead on health-related issues, while the public accounts committee or the like would take the lead on fiscal-related issues and how the plan takes all relevant issues into account.

The government and legislature also have an important role in ensuring that public health legislation and emergency powers legislation allow sufficient scope for public health decrees, lockdowns, and command over resources to produce essential health-related products during a pandemic.

6. Governance Challenges Especially During a Pandemic

Although what we propose for governance for pandemic preparation is not perfect, it should go a long way to having a government and public health system that is well prepared for a pandemic. When a pandemic arises, however, the executive branch of government and the public health

---

[35] In the lead-up to the Global Financial Crisis, many U.S. and European regulators and governments did not have the will to act against growing financial instability. In particular, they did not require financial institutions to have significantly more capital to buffer potential losses, especially related to loans and securities where there had been significant financial innovation, as in those related to residential mortgages.

agencies will need to take the decisions, subject to certain actions needing the approval of the appropriate legislature. As in pandemic preparation, the will to act (especially at the beginning of a pandemic) will be extremely important. Delay can lead to a rapid acceleration in the number of cases and deaths. Groupthink can sometimes be the cause of delay, so leaders need to listen intently to those voices arguing for quick action.

In crisis management of pandemics, there are some key actions that need to be taken to minimize significant errors.[36] These include active oversight by the president (or prime minister) of responses by all government department and agencies, and preparation for a crisis that is worse than currently expected. This preparation may, at times, require contemplating "war-time-like" command over the inputs for, and production of, key health-related goods.

In this section, we lay out some of the challenges that will be faced by governments during a pandemic (6.1). We then discuss what actions prior to the pandemic will increase the likelihood that good decisions will be made (6.2).

6.1 *Bureaucratic and political impediments to effective governance*

Bureaucratic inertia and/or poor organizational design can frustrate implementation of recommendations. As well, groupthink can get in the way of responding appropriately to new information. A potentially more dangerous problem is deliberate bureaucratic and/or political obfuscation that frustrates reforms in an attempt to shift blame for failures in a crisis. And, finally, a pandemic, with poor preparation and rushed policies, can be exploited by the unscrupulous in the private and public sectors for financial, political, or bureaucratic advantage. We will explore all three problems.

6.1.1 *Bureaucratic inertia and poor organizational design*

Our earlier discussion provides examples of organization inertia where reviews and suggested reforms have been placed on low priority or ignored. This may be not from any desire to avoid issues, but because the

---

[36] These ideas benefitted from private correspondence from Paul Tucker.

reforms were placed on a lower priority due to more pressing demands. It is tempting to ignore or downplay low-frequency, high-cost events by arguing that they will not happen in the foreseeable future.

6.1.2 *Deliberate bureaucratic and political obfuscation*

The impediment of deliberate bureaucratic and political obfuscation is potentially far more dangerous and costly. Given a pandemic or major event, there will be examples of failures that can be detected with hindsight. A well-functioning organization will prepare the political and media systems for possible failures given the inherent uncertainties of new pandemics. The correct approach is to admit uncertainties as they unfold, explaining any errors as they occur, including prompt remedial actions.

The worst response is to not admit errors, abuse honest critics, and try to cover up failure. This is not a sensible long-term strategy as invariably with investigative reporters, leaks, etc., the truth will out. Then, officialdom and their political masters compound error with lying. This destroys public trust which is difficult to remedy.

6.1.3 *A case study of political and bureaucratic failure and obfuscation*[37]

In Australia, the State government of Victoria has presided over a COVID policy and implementation crisis. The facts are as follows:

1. Until June 2020, Australia through rigorous quarantine and border entry restrictions had very limited COVID infections and deaths.[38]
2. The Australian Federal government had offered all the states defense personnel to act as hotel security for international arrivals. The Victorian state government declined the offer.

---

[37] Some of the material in this case study is taken from the following media sources: https://www.theguardian.com/australia-news/2020/nov/06/victorian-hotel-quarantine-inquiry-calls-for-police-to-be-on-site-24-hours-a-day; https://www.youtube.com/watch?v=QKxrfVYOfzI&list=PL2OFHLSeLxlbGzt7FOq8P2SE9GJajLYKh.

[38] See https://www.worldometers.info/coronavirus/country/australia/.

3. The Victorian state government in a hurried decision employed a private security firm to act as security personnel in the Melbourne quarantine hotels. The security firm was not on the prescribed list and a subsequent inquiry could not determine who made this decision.[39]

4. Subsequently, some arrivals infected the private security personnel, who in turn infected Melbourne citizens. There were allegations that the security firm employees had minimal training for their quarantine security tasks.

5. A Victorian COVID-19 hotel quarantine inquiry observed in November 2020 that 99% of the more than 20,000 cases and over 800 deaths related to COVID-19 in Victoria since late May could be traced back to the outbreaks among staff and security guards at the hotels. By December 2020, Australia had just over 900 deaths, with 820 in Victoria. Nearly all Victorian infections and deaths were in the greater Melbourne region.[40]

6. An additional failing was the lack of adequate preparation in long-term care homes. By mid-June there was ample international evidence that long-term care homes were major risk centers for COVID infections. The existing structure was a tragedy waiting to happen. A majority of the Melbourne deaths were in long-term care homes.[41]

7. Subsequent media investigations alleged that the state government did not follow due process in hiring the security firm. A senior bureaucrat and a minister resigned.

8. The State government imposed a very restrictive lockdown in Melbourne, resulting in serious economic and social costs. The state has had its debt rating downgraded as a result of the large fiscal deficits sustained during the lockdowns.[42]

---

[39] There has been a Victorian COVID-19 hotel quarantine inquiry that reported late December 2020. See https://www.parliament.vic.gov.au/file_uploads/0387_RC_Covid-19_Final_Report_Volume_1_v21_Digital_77QpLQH8.pdf.

[40] See https://covidlive.com.au/states-and-territories and https://covidlive.com.au/vic/postcode.

[41] See the discussion in the Lancet. https://www.thelancet.com/action/showPdf?pii=S0140-6736%2820%2932206-6.

[42] See https://www.abc.net.au/news/2020-12-07/victoria-loses-its-aaa-credit-rating-after-s&p-downgrades-state/12957626 and https://www.afr.com/policy/economy/victoria-s-credit-rating-downgraded-moody-s-20210223-p57517.

To summarize, this disaster showed serious policy and implementation errors, bordering on incompetence.

6.1.4 *Corruption*[43]

Whenever there are major government decisions that require large increases in expenditure and procurement, there are increased incentives for political and bureaucratic corruption. These incentives are magnified when policies are introduced in haste, and the usual safeguards and protocols are under stress. There may be good reasons why protocols that are appropriate for normal times cannot be followed because the risk of the costs of waiting to procure needed equipment or to make decisions based on the timelines implicit in normal protocols outweighs the risk of not making the best decision (when viewed ex post).

These implications of any major crisis that involves hurried large increases in expenditure should be anticipated. A pandemic is just an example of a major crisis. As the COVID crisis finally comes under control, and the costs are counted in health, social, and economic consequences, there will be increasing allegations of corruption at various levels. For example, financial support to firms or workers can be misdirected either because they have been rolled out in haste, exploited using loopholes, or are straight out fraud. In some jurisdictions where political corruption is more common, a crisis provides opportunities for large-scale fraud and embezzlement. Jurisdictions with high-quality audits should reveal the extent of these costs.

To reduce the costs of excess public expenditure due to fraud and related activities, planning should include developing information systems, protocols, and procedures that reduce these costs.

6.2 *Minimizing the failure to meet the challenges*

Good preparation, along the lines we laid out, should minimize the chances that governments will fall into traps presented by the challenges

---

[43]This section draws upon, https://images.transparencycdn.org/images/Getting-ahead-of-the-curve.pdf; https://www.transparency.org/en/press/open-letter-to-the-g20-finance-ministers.

we have analyzed, as well as other challenges that may be thrown up as a pandemic progresses. The following are key to these preparations:

- A clear plan that is frequently updated and that includes outside-the-box thinking where appropriate.
- Regular training regarding a plan for personnel, including senior bureaucrats and ministers, that stresses the importance of acting early in a pandemic to prevent its rapid spread.[44]
- An independent agency to evaluate regularly and frequently whether the plan is being followed.
- Legislative committees that review postmortems, plans, and evaluations and hold the government to account.

In Chapter 5, we will add another key element of being ready to meet challenges: the regular use of stress tests and exercises (wargames), including the participation of senior personnel.

7. Conclusion

There has been a clear lack of preparation by many countries in dealing with the COVID-19 virus epidemic. The resultant economic and social costs have been very large. Policy decisions were taken under considerable uncertainty about the virulence and lethality of the virus. The consequences of this uncertainty could have been reduced by better preparation.

We propose an expansion of private catastrophe risk insurance with a carefully crafted backstop to deal with major disasters that are beyond the capacity of private insurance companies. This organization can draw on

---

[44] Michael Lewis (2021) discusses the inertia of the Centers for Disease Control (CDC) and the Trump administration at the beginning of the COVID-19 pandemic in the U.S. The CDC appears to have been affected by groupthink and a belief that it could never risk having restrictions that *ex post* would turn out to have been too tight, given its experience in an earlier episode.

the insurance industries' personnel, as well as databases accumulated in their property and business interruption business.

Good governance, with an appropriate degree of independence for agencies and effective legislative committees, can increase the probability that pandemic preparation, including appropriate postmortems, plans, and implementation of plans, can be well done. Good postmortems and plans are a prerequisite for running the types of appropriate stress tests and exercises (wargames) that we discuss in the next chapter.

References

Box, G. E. (1976). "Science and Statistics," *Journal of the American Statistical Association*, 71(356), December, 791–799.

Carney, M. (2021). *Value (s): Building a Better World for All*. Signal Books, New York.

Chowell *et al.* (2016). https://www.ncbi.nlm.nih.gov/pmc/articles/PMC5348083/.

Crean, J. and Milne, F. (2022). "Covid and Other Catastrophes — Systemic Risks Neglected by Financial System Reform," Working Paper forthcoming.

Green, T. (2021). *The Covid Consensus: The New Politics of Global Inequality*. Hurst and Company, London.

Kirchhoff (2020). https://www.statnews.com/2020/03/24/chris-kirchhoff-ebola-coronavirus-response/.

Lewis, M. (2021). *The Premonition*. Norton and Company, New York.

The New York Times (2020). https://int.nyt.com/data/documenthelper/6824-2019-10-key-findings-and-after/05bd797500ea55be0724/optimized/full.pdf.

Tucker, P. (2018). *Unelected Power: The Quest for Legitimacy in Central Banking and the Regulatory State*. Princeton University Press, New Jersey.

Chapter 5

Pandemic Preparedness

1. Introduction

There is an important interdependence between economic, financial, and health policy actions. The recent COVID-19 crisis has demonstrated that, apart from the direct economic consequences from illness and death from the virus, the main economic, financial, and social costs have been due to the varying degrees of preventative measures taken by the public, firms, and governments that directly impacted economic and financial activity.

In attempts to ameliorate the impact on the welfare of the population, governments have taken major interventions in real and financial markets. These policies can be very expensive, of varying degrees of effectiveness, and can have major implications for the size of increases in unemployment, government deficits, and debt levels.[1] The economic, social, and fiscal implications of strong lockdown, more focused quarantine policies, and all the variations in between require careful analysis, incorporating those lessons into stress tests and wargames.

---

[1] For an analysis of the economic and social consequences of widespread lockdown policies by many countries, see Green (2021). Major concerns have been a significant increase in social and economic inequality induced by lockdown policies disrupting economic activity and the education of children. Especially concerning are the implications for children and the poor in the Global South.

The declines in national GDP over 2020 were dramatic (as were sub-sequent rapid recoveries).[2] Fiscal responses to subsidize sectors hard hit by lockdown policies saw unprecedented peacetime government deficits and commensurate increases in government debt.[3]

In this chapter, we explore new methods in planning and preparing for such major events. They are designed to reduce the likelihood and severity of the health and economic costs of a pandemic. These general planning methods have been used in the past as risk management tools in both the health and financial fields, but they have not so far been considered as an integrated system. In particular, we describe the use of integrated stress tests and exercises (or wargames) to prepare for a future pandemic.[4]

Various versions of stress tests have been used widely in the financial sector, particularly after the Global Financial Crisis (GFC) of 2007–2009 during which the lesson learned was that they were not stressful enough. Wargames have been used to prepare for extreme events that will stretch health, economic, social, physical, and organizational resources. But, there has been a major weakness in that these exercises have been played within sectors, but not across sectors. The key recommendation of this chapter is that systemic wargames be played regularly to prepare for pandemics and other major societal disruptions.

The outline of this chapter is as follows: Section 2 describes the methodology of financial stress tests that have been used for individual banks and the banking system. We describe financial stress tests used before the GFC, their development, and their widespread use after the GFC. We explore the limitations of this methodology.

Section 3 discusses the methodology and conduct of pandemic exercises that had been implemented in the past. These games had a similar methodology to financial stress tests and suffered from comparable

---

[2] For example, the UK Office for Budge Responsibility has issued a report estimating the fall in GDP in various countries from COVID lockdown policies. See Chart 2 page 5 in https://obr.uk/frr/fiscal-risks-report-july-2021/.

[3] See Chapter 2 in https://obr.uk/frr/fiscal-risks-report-july-2021/.

[4] In this chapter, we will refer to wargames. In the health literature, they are often referred to as exercises. Effectively, they are the same procedure. A stress test is a more limited operation which describes a scenario and explores its direct consequences. The differences between wargames and stress tests will be discussed in more detail as follows.

limitations. In addition, as we observed in Chapter 4, they had other major limitations including the absence of analysis of social, economic, financial, and fiscal implications of policy options.

In Section 4, we argue that wargame methodology, combined with improved pandemic models, should improve policy responses in the health and government sectors.

Section 5 discusses lessons learned from our recent experience with the COVID-19 pandemic, and relates them to stress testing and wargames.

Section 6 proposes a serious program of wargame preparation for future pandemics. These exercises would integrate health, social, economic, financial, and fiscal sectors to test systems and policy strategies. In addition, these exercises provide an important educative and training role for decision-makers and key employees in these sectors.

The chapter concludes with Section 7, which is a summary with policy recommendations.

2. Financial Stress Testing

2.1 *The history and methodology of stress tests*[5]

Stress tests have a long history in engineering where structures are tested for their durability under extreme conditions. The idea has been adapted in banks and other financial institutions where stress testing refers to modeling exercises where extreme events are used to test for the size of losses in trading, credit, or other areas of the institution.

A stress test for a bank begins by outlining a financial and economic scenario which implies losses in the trading and credit books of the bank. The aim of the exercise is to estimate the potential losses due to such a scenario. Banks will try various scenarios over time, adjusting the scenarios that they think are possible but have a low subjective likelihood. The scenarios will often use empirical data or experience from previous crises. This methodology was widely used in the banking sector before the

---

[5] See Dent, Westwood, and Segoviano (2016) for an excellent introduction to stress testing methodology.

GFC, but its use was limited to particular sections of banking operations and rarely as bank-wide, integrated tests.

Before the 2007–2009 GFC, most bank stress tests were conducted within the banks themselves, with few being done by regulators. An exception was the IMF; in its five-year Financial Sector Assessment Program examinations, it had begun to use stress test scenarios in 1999 following the 1997 Asian Financial Crisis.[6] Since the crisis, regulators have conducted stress tests at a couple of levels: at the individual bank level and, in some cases, simultaneously across banks.

The GFC provided strong evidence of failures in many standard risk management practices. The failures occurred in both the private sector, particularly in banks with weak risk management systems, and the regulatory system.

2.2 *Risk management practices and the GFC*

2.2.1 *GFC failures in risk management and subsequent innovations*[7]

Risk managers and financial regulators have long grappled with the limitations of modeling financial markets, credit, liquidity, and systemic risks.[8] Before the GFC, risk management models were regarded as being accurate, protecting banks from major losses. For example, market risks are the risks that investment banks and trading arms of commercial banks were exposed to in their financial trading operations. These trading operations were based on theoretical and statistical models that required strong assumptions to calculate price and hedging strategies.

Model limitations were described as model risk. Different models were used to try to deal with real complexity. Astute risk managers attached to trading floors were constantly back-testing models for

---

[6] See https://www.imf.org/external/pubs/ft/fandd/2019/09/what-is-stress-testing-basics.htm.

[7] This section draws upon Milne (2008) and (2009).

[8] See Dowd (2005) for a text book discussion. For a more general discussion of risk management modeling used before the GFC, see Crouhy, Mark, and Galai (2000).

accuracy by observing outcomes. Using experience and knowing the limitations of specific models were crucial to avoid large trading losses. The models rely on important parameters that can only be estimated with error. Therefore, the models should have been run with a range of plausible parameter estimates to detect possible hedging losses. The risks associated with parameter estimation were described as estimation risks.

One of the major errors that risk managers can make is to rely solely on models that seem to work well in "normal times," where price movements are relatively small and described by well-known stochastic process models and their estimated parameters. But, if there are major disruptions with large price movements, especially when different asset prices, rather than moving independently, begin to move together, normal-time hedging strategies can fail dramatically with large losses. An additional concern is that hedging strategies that rely on liquid markets can discover that, in a crisis, markets can become "thin" so that trading even at normal levels will move prices against the trader, and, in extreme cases, it will be difficult to find traders on the other side of the trade. This lack of functioning markets in key financial assets can destroy hedging strategies, creating heavy losses for banks and other institutions.

Another example revealed in the GFC was the misuse of credit and trading models, especially for mortgage-backed securities. In the lead-up to the GFC, housing markets in key areas of the US, Ireland, and some other countries showed all the signs of an asset bubble, with poor credit underwriting standards on many mortgages. When the real estate markets peaked in 2006 and began to fall in 2007, the losses appeared in derivatives whose asset prices reflected the failing mortgages. By the middle of 2007, the market losses began to work their way through the financial markets, until the magnitude of the losses became apparent on the balance sheets of major banks and financial institutions around the world.[9]

One technique that attempts to address the problems inherent in model and estimation risk is to use stress tests. A financial model stress test imposes an extreme scenario using either past data or constructed data

---

[9]The insurance company IAG had a large business insuring defaults on mortgage-backed securities. Using flawed models, IAG suffered huge losses when mortgage defaults increased dramatically.

to test the accuracy and reliability of the models. This can be extended to models in related areas in the bank to check for interactions in trading and credit strategies, checking for potential large losses.

During the GFC, it became obvious that some banks had been prudent in their use of models, understanding their limitations and acting to remedy deficiencies. Other banks had been imprudent and suffered accordingly.

Given below is a summary[10]:

(a) Back-testing is standard practice in attempting to validate models. Many models show their limitations in back-tests, especially in extreme market conditions.
(b) Stressed market conditions are extremely difficult to predict with statistical models. Data are often sparse and non-stationary, so that model predictions often lack statistical robustness.
(c) To complement the statistical models used for "normal" times, stress tests — or, in some limited cases, financial wargames — are widely used to consider the effects of extreme downside outcomes.

2.2.2 Concurrent financial stress tests run by regulators[11]

A more ambitious stress test used by regulators is a concurrent stress test where the regulators present several banks under their jurisdiction with the same scenario. The banks will each use the scenario to run their own stress tests independently. Then, the regulator checks the results comparing how each bank fares, looking for inconsistencies or weaknesses within and across banks' balance sheets and income statements.

Stress tests play an important role checking for weaknesses in the banking system and educating risk managers and regulators. These tests begin by postulating a scenario where there are weaknesses in the real

---

[10] The methodological modeling issues that we saw in pandemic models reappear in financial risk management models: data limitations, model choices, strategic choices impacting outcomes, etc.

[11] This is a complex topic, and we will merely sketch the main points. For a detailed discussion of this material, see the report by the BIS (2017).

economy (e.g., a significant fall in GDP, a rise in unemployment, and a major fall in asset prices). Given this scenario, the test then estimates the consequences for bank losses and potential insolvencies. It is important that the stress tests be used constructively so that any bank weaknesses can be rectified promptly.

Although they are a very useful tool for risk management, stress tests have a number of well-known weaknesses. We will mention three of the most important as follows:

(a) Stress tests rely heavily on models of assets returns and credit losses. As noted earlier, these models can be quite reliable in "normal" times where the data fall well in the range of past observations: The distribution of returns can be estimated with some confidence. But, in a stress test scenario, the asset returns will be from the extreme tail of the assumed probability distribution; correlations can change dramatically, so that the estimates of returns in the scenario will lack statistical significance.[12]

(b) Stress tests of a single bank do not consider the impact of a single bank's insolvency on the rest of the banking system, where losses are transmitted through the interbank market. Some central banks use top-down models of bank networks to consider solvency issues that arise in interbank markets.[13]

(c) A weakness of the basic top-down network model is that it does not allow for bank reactions in trading, adjusting their assets and liabilities when reacting to a severe economic and/or financial scenario. Central bank models have attempted to accommodate this criticism of their network models by appending liquidity modules that allow for price movements induced by large asset trades by banks in the

---

[12] For a detailed analysis and strong critique of modeling issues in concurrent stress tests by the US Federal Reserve and the Bank of England, see Dowd (2014, 2016); and Buckner and Dowd (2021) for the recent COVID-19 stress test.

[13] For example, see the Bank of England's RAMSI model described in Burrows, Learmonth, McKeown, and Williams (2012).

network.[14] Given the complexity of this modification, it requires a number of modeling shortcuts that are not entirely satisfactory.

Another approach that exploits agent interactions and reduces the heavy reliance of models is to use wargames. Although these wargames often use modeling as an input, their use requires understanding of their limitations. This is where specialists in various areas who play the game provide professional experience and judgment that models can seldom achieve.

3. Previous Pandemic Exercises

In Chapters 2 and 4, we discussed examples of pandemic reports and exercises that were performed before the current pandemic. Some of these exercises appeared to be perfunctory, while others were much more elaborate. There are many examples where the recommendations from the exercises were ignored by authorities.[15] Prior to the COVID-19 pandemic, strong lockdown policies were not recommended by many epidemiologists who cited the social and economic costs of strong lockdown policy.[16] We suspect this is the reason that pre-COVID pandemic exercises ignored social and economic consequences of these strong policy actions.

As a consequence, there had been no attempt to integrate the lessons from the GFC and the medical wargames prior to the COVID-19 crisis. It has become obvious that many of the policies attempting to reduce the spread of the virus have had very significant negative social, economic, financial, and fiscal consequences. There have been far too many cases where decision-makers have been ill prepared for dealing with the various consequences of their policy actions. For decision-makers to have a better

---

[14] For example, see the discussion of the Bank of Canada's MFRAF model in Fique (2017).

[15] See Carney (2021) Chapter 9 for a strong critique of the lack of preparation.

[16] Analysis of strong lockdowns versus more targeted quarantine policies has become an ongoing, highly charged debate in the media and social media. The introduction of COVID vaccines has further complicated this policy debate. We hope that careful, dispassionate analysis of the evidence, after the pandemic subsides, will provide insights on appropriate policies.

understanding of the consequences of various policy options, we advocate the implementation of regular, integrated wargames that test these aspects of a pandemic.

4. Background on Wargames

4.1 *History and methodology of military games*

Wargaming was used professionally in the German Army from the middle of the 19th Century. Other armies quickly copied the ideas — for a history, see Thomas Allen (1987), (2015) and more recently Hershkovitz (2019).[17] Wargames are also known as Simulations or Exercises. They all share a common methodology.

There are three basic forms of wargames:

(a) Table-top wargames with figures, counters, etc. Civilian versions are Chess, Diplomacy, Risk, or far more sophisticated computer game versions. Strategic computer wargames played by civilians are often spin-offs of Pentagon wargames.
(b) Field exercises using real troops and equipment.
(c) Large-scale strategic games using computer simulations and predictive models (NATO Wargames are a good example). Typically, these games have two sides (the Red enemy and the Blue home nation). There can be many players, allies, etc. The games allow sophisticated play using intelligence evaluations of enemy and allied policies.

4.2 *The history and methodology of corporate wargames*

Corporate wargaming has been used for some time. For an excellent summary of the pitfalls and advantages, see Horn (2011).[18] These games incorporate strategic scenarios that try to avoid the simplifications and ambiguities (multiple equilibria) of models based on game theory.

---

[17] See Curry and Drage (2020) for a handbook of cyber attacks and wargames with a number of worked examples.
[18] Horn (2011).

Wargames go far beyond mathematical predictive models by incorporating the judgment and experience of professionals with detailed knowledge of various functions of complex organizations.

The game design is critical for meaningful learning. The game should help in analyzing corporate problems. This involves careful analysis of corporate financial and legal procedures, regulatory interactions, and the strategic interactions of competitors. The game design should decide whether to concentrate on narrow tactical and procedural scenarios or more general scenarios. This will determine the type of players (experience and relevance) involved. Games should be repeated with different but Plausible Worse-Case (PWC) scenarios. This is a learning experience for decision-makers who in a real crisis will have to make major decisions — often under considerable uncertainty and severe pressure in real time.

4.3 *Government and policy relevant wargames*

Government (civilian) wargames follow the same general methodology, as explained in the McKinsey report (Horn, 2011), but can be far more complex in dealing with multiple institutions in the context of strategic, economic, health, financial, and other emergencies.[19] From history, we know that low-probability/high-cost (in the broadest sense) events resonate through the social and economic system, often inducing major problems and having long-run consequences for the private, public, and political sectors.

Private sector and government policy responses can amplify or dampen the impact of the initial event: Poorly prepared governments can amplify the impact — often with dire long-term implications. This implies that policy responses require careful analysis of possible "unintended consequences." These consequences are important for designing the appropriate responses, conditional on the best information available at any time. Furthermore, strategies should be considered to be conditional on new information, so actions can adapt. Approaching strategic planning using this approach requires careful analysis so that adequate preparation

---

[19] For an early grand political/diplomatic/economic/financial wargame, see Kubarych (2001).

is built into policy responses. Human and physical resources and their organization take time to build, so that lack of preparation in a crisis will induce costly actions and mistakes that could have been avoided.

Policy-relevant wargames are an important tool in preparing for these types of extreme events. They should be a normal method of planning responses to low-probability high-cost events, and *not* an optional extra.

One important component in any wargame exercise is the use of lessons learned from previous extreme events. Detailed forensic reports from previous crises should be used as guides in constructing scenarios and exploring strategies.

4.4 *Wargame analysis: Cognitive limitations*[20]

The role of a wargame is not to predict the future, but to explore various plausible worst-case scenarios. The game requires experts, decision-makers, and other players to interact and learn from the experience. Games are most productive when conventional or standard responses are found wanting, so that the players can experiment, trying novel solutions to problems without imposing heavy costs in real time due to a flawed strategy.

An additional benefit is that standard ways of thinking about problems, group think, and other cognitive biases can be challenged. This learning experience should be used to foster innovation in the structure of the organization, updating procedures, and equipment. The games should be used to challenge complacency: An emergency that occurred many years ago may have engendered procedures and equipment that have become obsolete, given current knowledge and technology. A well-designed game can reveal those weaknesses.

If the games are played regularly, then key players will become familiar with the other players and their skills. This familiarity reduces the risk of player conflict and misunderstandings in a real crisis when time pressure and stress can lead to confusion, poor decision-making, and flawed implementation.

---

[20]This discussion draws on Hershkovitz (2019), particularly pp. 10–14.

4.5 *How do we use wargame results?*

The results and lessons learned from games should be written up and used to revise plans (and manuals), and implemented by changing organizations and procedures. Although military and strategic wargame results and briefing notes are top secret,[21] there is no good reason why pandemic and other environmental wargame results should be secret. The results should be carefully communicated to major players and experts in the private and public sectors for discussion. The discussions and feedback can be used in later rounds of wargames, improving organizational and response strategies.

Wargames are excellent educational exercises for major players who will be involved in low-probability/high-cost events. Public sectors in the related areas should be involved in planning and playing a game.

A crucial part of the wargame exercise is a serious review to ensure that reforms or actions recommended in the report have been implemented within 6 to 12 months. Otherwise, the game and resulting report of what was learned in the wargame are just an expensive waste of time, ignored and filed to gather dust. The public dissemination of wargames and their results is a critical part of the wargame process. Open discussion and evaluation are important as an educational exercise.

4.6 *Starting points for systemic wargame playing: Two Canadian examples*

We argue that with sufficient preparation with stress tests, wargaming, and improved information systems, estimates of economic losses and social impacts across sectors can be improved. This should allow more targeted and effective policy strategies. There may be extreme situations that are very difficult to wargame as they lie outside even the most thoughtful and creative policy planners. Wargaming is not a panacea, but a serious tool to be applied by planners.

Systemic wargames should be adapted to cover environmental and other systemic risks. To illustrate this argument, we discuss two Canadian

---

[21] See Allen (2015).

examples of starting points for wargames. We emphasize that these examples are starting points for more extensive wargames that we are advocating.

4.6.1 *Example 1: A major Vancouver earthquake*

The Le Pan study,[22] imagining a major earthquake in Vancouver, British Columbia, provides a detailed analysis of the implications for the insurance industry, coinsurance, and ultimately the key role of Government funding back-stops. A major earthquake would lead to severe damage to commercial and domestic real estate. Insurance companies would face major claims. Some of the claims would have been reinsured on the international market, but the amounts could be so large, the British Columbia Provincial and Canadian Federal governments would find it necessary to provide financial subsidies to the insurance companies.

Rather than face ex-post actions, a well-prepared system of risk management would have the appropriate medical, civil engineering, financial, and economic procedures in place and tested regularly. There should be government contracts that stipulate conditional payments that insurance companies and banks can use in their stress tests. In the case of banks, major damage, disruption of economic activity, and stress on financial balance sheets will impact credit risks. Bank lending policies would take these contracts into account.[23]

Although most households in British Columbia have earthquake insurance, other vulnerable regions of Canada are underinsured for major earthquakes. Federal and provincial government actuarial analysis should take these systemic risks into account.

A major Vancouver earthquake would not just create destruction of real estate properties but it would also disrupt local and national commerce, especially as Vancouver is the Pacific port for Canadian–Asian trade. These effects should be wargamed, as the cost and disruptions can be subtle, creating major systemic losses that, to the unprepared, will appear surprising.

---

[22] Our discussion here draws upon Le Pan (2016).

[23] See Le Pan (2016) and Crean and Milne (2022) for a detailed analysis.

4.6.2 *Example 2: The Ontario SARS pandemic experience*

The Ontario SARS Report, which we referred to in Chapter 4,[24] should have been used as the basis for routine major wargames on pandemics that would test not only the health system but also the related economic and financial systems, that would be impacted by various quarantine strategies of increasing severity. It should have been obvious that so-called lockdown policies and associated socially disruptive policies would have major implications for economic, financial, and social activity.

The key players should have detailed playbooks for systemic environmental, pandemic, and other events. These playbooks would be useful guides and invaluable for training regulators, politicians, and senior management in the private and public sectors. But, recent reports indicate that such games were not played. Indeed, many of the SARS Report recommendations were not implemented.

5. Lessons from the COVID-19 Crisis

The pandemic has revealed many flaws in the health system. These are hard lessons that should be incorporated into future planning and wargames. We discuss health, economic, and financial consequences directly caused by the pandemic and by policies implemented to combat the virus.

5.1 *Health lessons from the COVID-19 crisis*

The COVID-19 pandemic evolved rapidly with increasing discussion of appropriate policy responses. The results of the Crimson Contagion game, the Kirchhoff Report, and other wargames were useful guides pointing to the failures in national health responses. There were serious discussions by epidemiologists concerning weaknesses and omissions in current medical data on comorbidity rates, mild/unreported infections, and their impact on estimated mortality rates, etc. In turn, this resulted in a professional debate on the predictive power of pandemic models that were used

---

[24] See SARS Commission Report, Ontario (2008).

in the early months of the crisis. Some models had major problems predicting the course of the virus and its fatality rates. For example, some models did not allow for population behavioral changes, where people became more cautious, distancing, wearing masks in crowded environments, etc. These modeling and predictive limitations added to the uncertainty over the choice of appropriate responses to the virus.[25] Subsequently, there have been advances in modeling the spread of the virus and fatality rates, using more disaggregated data and modeling strategies. These developments are very welcome.[26]

The health sector has come under serious stress with increased workloads in key areas. Resources have been switched from lower-priority areas to pandemic-related areas. These areas were constrained in the short run because specialized capacity took time to adapt. For example, there were shortages of protective clothing, surgical masks, ventilators, and other equipment. Supplies of critical drugs, testing kits, and physical equipment have been in very short supply, requiring rapid increases in production, sometimes from non-standard suppliers.

Vaccine development and production take time: Traditional vaccine methods required years of development, requiring careful testing for effectiveness and serious side effects to gain regulatory approval. With the onset of the pandemic, newer mRNA vaccines were fast-tracked in emergency programs. Early in the pandemic, authorities were unsure when effective vaccines would be available for mass vaccinations. Uncertainty over the timing, effectiveness, and availability of a vaccine is critical in developing strategic responses. Wargames should explore various scenarios where vaccines become available early or late in a pandemic. These expectations will have a major impact on strategies, trading off the possible timeliness and effectiveness of a vaccine against prolonged lockdown policies or other strategies. As it turned out, by the end of 2020, a number of pharmaceutical companies were producing vaccines based on

---

[25] See Adam (2020) and https://www.economist.com/graphic-detail/2020/05/23/early-projections-of-covid-19-in-america-underestimated-its-severity.

[26] For example, see Ellison (2020).

the relatively new technology of mRNA.[27] It will be important to monitor the effectiveness of mRNA vaccines in guarding against other diseases, so as to update estimates on how quickly an mRNA vaccine for another coronavirus pandemic could be developed for a new virus. It will also be important to monitor the production capacity for mRNA and other vaccines and to consider steps to augment that capacity if a future pandemic occurs.

There have been strong incentives to slow the spread of the virus by distancing rules, masking, testing, quarantine, and/or the more severe lockdown regulations. Some countries and regions had their health systems severely stressed, while many other regions had idle pandemic medical capacity.

Ongoing data analysis is trying to identify key economic, demographic, and geographic variables that explain these variations. Some authorities have asserted that a hard lockdown was the optimal strategy.[28] But, this strategy is open to question, given the experience of some regions or countries with lower death rates, which did not implement a full lockdown strategy, using a more targeted quarantine and testing strategy.[29] Some countries used a combination of aggressive testing and intermediate restrictions concentrating on sections of the population that were most vulnerable.[30]

---

[27] For a history of this technology, see https://www.nature.com/articles/nrd.2017.243 and, for its rapid development during the COVID pandemic, see https://www.uab.edu/news/youcanuse/item/12059-covid-19-mrna-vaccines-how-could-anything-developed-this-quickly-be-safe.

[28] Lockdown is a generic name for a range of quarantine policies of varying degrees of severity. Media reports often do not discriminate between the various policies, leading to public confusion.

[29] For example, see Germany, South Korea, Japan, and Taiwan. Within the USA, the highly varied experience of different states will require careful study, exploring quarantine and testing strategies, demographics, time of onset of the epidemic, etc. See this site for USA state data, https://www.worldometers.info/coronavirus/country/us/.

[30] Japan, South Korea, and Taiwan are examples using this strategy in 2020. It is important to note that these countries had previous experience with viruses that emanated from China. They appear to have been well prepared. Careful study of these countries' policies and experiences with the COVID-19 virus would be prudent.

It has become apparent in many countries that lack of testing and the availability of appropriate tests hampered a clear evaluation of the virulence and lethality for various demographic groups. In early 2020, a number of eminent epidemiologists had questioned the quality and interpretation of existing data used to inform policy.[31]

5.2 *Communication lessons from the COVID-19 crisis*

Many governments made statements that lockdowns would last for many months, and/or there could be a series of lockdowns. Such unconditional statements ignored the high uncertainty relating to the spread of the pandemic and the lethality/virulence of the virus. The evolution of knowledge and appropriate data can make unconditional statements obsolete within a few days, diminishing respect for the integrity and competence of government policy.

Changes in information and confusion about the reality of the pandemic and policies should be incorporated into exercise/wargames. For example, as the COVID-19 epidemic spread, more accurate data and testing had revealed patterns that have allowed more targeted responses and reduced the worst fears of massive numbers of deaths. Prior to the approval of vaccines, deaths appear to be overwhelmingly concentrated in the very elderly and those with immune deficiencies.

There has been public confusion over cases revealed by widespread testing and the likelihood of death due to COVID. Much of the (social and mainstream) media and many governments have created widespread fear by emphasizing COVID cases without indicating whether the case was asymptomatic, required hospitalization, or resulted in death. It was well-known by June 2020 that COVID severity was strongly related to age and comorbidities: Announcing "cases" without the important qualifications spread alarm in the public.

Fears have also been exaggerated by quoting raw number of cases and deaths without placing them in context, in relation to total population numbers, or in comparison to normal death rates in society. Conspiracy theories and misinformation have confused the public. Many governments have had poor

---

[31] For example, see Roussel *et al.* (2020) and Ioannidis (2020).

communication policies, adding to the confusion. And, in some extreme cases, governments have exploited public fears for electoral advantage, or to introduce powers beyond what would be regarded a commensurate with the risks.

Similar communication problems have arisen in public and media discussion of various medical treatments and vaccination. Social media has compounded the problem where misinformation and conspiracy theories are legion. These sources of information thrive on apparent contradictory public health statements. Statements or policies that were based on information at some prior date are ridiculed later when more refined information has become available. It is critical that policy statements be prefaced with a strong emphasis that they are made conditional on the best information at the time. Furthermore, it should be made clear that future policies will be adjusted to accommodate new information.

5.3 *Economic lessons from the COVID-19 crisis*

Lockdown policies extending over months severely stressed social, economic, and financial systems in a profound and complex manner.

To understand those consequences, one requires detailed microeconomic and institutional analyses. Partial equilibrium economic models help in evaluating industry impact. But, there are profound systemic effects that require explicit or implicit general equilibrium analysis. This analysis requires ex-ante and ex-post tactics and policies that are go far beyond conventional — and inadequate — macroeconomic and financial macroprudential policy analysis. Economic research should explore theoretical and empirical models and data collection that provides more accurate predictions for future pandemics.

For example, uncertainty about the length of the emergency measures substantially reduced consumer expenditures and firm sales as consumers and firms became increasingly cautious in their consumption and investment plans.[32] This prudence led to dramatic falls in some durable good

---

[32]Labor law also requires that employers have a safe workplace for their employees. Indeed, in Canada (and elsewhere) employees who believe their workplace is unsafe can refuse to work until it is inspected by the relevant authorities. Firms may also have legal risk if they are totally negligent in taking steps to ensure the safety of customers entering their premises. Given some firms and institutions have required employees to be vaccinated, labor laws should incorporate that possibility.

purchases, hospitality, travel, and firm investment. Unemployment rose rapidly to levels that far exceeded unemployment in the GFC.[33] Within months, it then declined sharply. These unemployment levels have obvious social and economic consequences.

Many governments have introduced large increases in current expenditure on social welfare payments, loans, and various employment subsidy schemes. These economic measures required governments to run large deficits, with commensurate dramatic increases in government debt. The expenditure and loan schemes have been put into place quickly, in many cases without adequate safeguards and preparation prior to the pandemic. In some cases, there will be unfortunate consequences:

(a) Obvious major anomalies in application will surface in future audits.
(b) The schemes will be more open to fraud than typical government programs because safeguards will be inadequate.
(c) By the time the schemes are fully operational, the main crisis may well have passed, so that expenditure may be inappropriately targeted before the schemes are wound down.
(d) Government loan schemes fed through banks create major conflicts with prudent credit procedures and bank supervisory rules. This is especially true for schemes that fail to discriminate between standard loans, simple wealth transfers, or combinations of both.[34]

Central banks used unconventional monetary policy to support fiscal policy and buffer the output and employment losses. This policy has often meant large increases in the central bank balance sheet and the risk of monetization of the increased government debt. Such monetization is

---

[33] Many countries have implemented employment subsidies which imply serious understatement of official unemployment figures. There should be clear data on temporary layoffs due to a lockdown versus longer-term unemployment. With repeated lockdowns, this distinction can become blurred.

[34] When loan officers are making credit decisions, they will consider government loans, querying the bank's priority in the list of creditors. For example, if the government loan is prior to the bank loan, then the bank loan will attract higher credit risk and a commensurate higher interest rate. Conversely, if the "loan" is a wealth transfer, that will reduce the credit risk of the bank loan, because some or all of it is automatically forgivable (or it is expected that in practice it is likely to be forgiven).

likely only in central banks which lack independence or are not committed to price stability.

Shutdowns and quarantines were instituted to contain the pandemic. Sectors of the economy were effectively graded from "essential" sectors through to "inessential" sectors. Inessential real sectors were partially or completely shut down by government fiat — these sectors suffered a collapse in revenue. They operated for weeks or months with drastically reduced operations, cutting employment and variable costs. Some firms in these sectors may never reopen. Shutdowns induced a dramatic increase in layoffs and unemployment as companies struggled to keep valued employees, unsure when they will be allowed to resume operations. Government agencies dealing with unemployment came under stress as they struggled with the increased workload. These consequences of lockdown policies need to be incorporated into the plans and contingencies prepared for fiscal and monetary policy.

Companies are restricted by their reserves of working capital. Banks have struggled to analyze extensions of credit given the uncertainty surrounding the length of time that government quarantine restrictions will be enforced, and the terms of government loans and subsidies.

Reductions in private sector activity worked their way through collapsing supply chains, retailing and wholesale sectors. While many inessential services largely shut down (such as travel, restaurants, sports, and culture), other sectors (such as distribution, online retailers, producers of recreational equipment, producers and supplies of goods and services related to home renovations, online entertainment, internet service, and IT business services) saw increased demand for their goods and services. This implied a dramatic redistribution of income and wealth within most economies.[35] To a large extent, losses were offset by various government subsidy schemes.

Given the speed of the evolution of the pandemic, and market reactions, governments have tried to keep pace with economic policies. Government departments have tried to obtain appropriate and timely data: In some cases, the data had not been collected or were difficult to collate

---

[35] For Canada, see https://www150.statcan.gc.ca/n1/pub/11-631-x/11-631-x2021001-eng.htm#a4 and internationally, https://www.imf.org/external/pubs/ft/fandd/2021/06/inequality-and-covid-19-ferreira.htm.

from various systems. There are the inevitable lags with bureaucracies struggling with new procedures and programs.

Attempts to predict which sectors would be badly impacted by lockdown policies have been hampered by the complexity of the modern economy. There are many subtle economic connections between different real and financial sectors of the economy and the labor force.

5.4   *Stressed domestic and international supply chains in the COVID-19 crisis*

Domestic supply chains were disrupted early in the crisis. Some products (e.g., food) were not, but manufactured products dependent on various component manufacturers suffered major or minor disruption. Disruption in a single key component can halt production of an end product. Just-in-time warehousing policies, designed to minimize normal time costs, are highly vulnerable to broad-based lockdown policies. International supply chains — largely originating in China — were disrupted for the first few months, but soon came back on stream.

How reliable these suppliers will be in future pandemics, in terms of providing the quantity and quality of goods ordered, is an open question, depending upon Chinese government policy and changes in Western government trade and strategic policies. More generally, there is a lively debate on the reliability of foreign suppliers, especially in key strategic commodities, e.g., pharmaceuticals, which are largely supplied by Chinese manufacturers.[36]

5.5   *Financial market responses in the COVID-19 pandemic*

Until early 2020, the US stock market had been regarded as overvalued by astute investors. Valuations had been boosted by the popularity of share buy-backs, resulting in increased leverage and elevated stock prices. Thus, valuations were highly sensitive to major declines in profits. Indeed, many

---

[36] See this June 2020 article in the Financial Times discussing the EU problems with international supply chain reliability, https://www.ft.com/content/af39c6d2-ae1e-4d0b-ba5b-121d12b22647.

of these highly levered companies saw heavy reductions in revenues and profits during the pandemic.

Stock market volatility in early 2020 increased dramatically, so that it replicated the worst period of the 2007–2009 crisis. The volatility was a result of continual revaluations driven by revelations about the disease, its prevalence, and death rates, as well as significant changes in information about the length of national lockdown strategies. Uncertainty about the length of the lockdown period, combined with many governments not being clear about conditions determining the length of the lockdown period, created increased uncertainty surrounding projections of future revenue, costs, and profits. In turn, this is factored into financial valuations of stocks, corporate bonds, and derivative securities.

By mid-2021, the US stock market indices greatly surpassed their pre-COVID level in early 2020. The US economy had largely recovered. But, the increased government expenditure by the US has been financed with greatly increased government debt and the Federal Reserve balance sheet. There has been considerable debate in financial markets about increases in inflation. The Federal Reserve claims that any price increases will be short-lived; others are less sanguine. Only time will tell.

Other countries in the EU (e.g., Italy) never recovered from the GFC, so that the economic cost associated with the pandemic has made their economies more fragile. These longer-term impacts will take time to work their way through the economic system.

Although stock market volatility is not necessarily a policy problem, it mirrored underlying market uncertainty in corporate cash flows stemming from government interventions. Furthermore, some countries, especially low-income ones, faced significant increases in sovereign risk premiums when issuing their government debt.

5.6 *The impact of COVID-19 on credit*

The GFC demonstrated the key role of credit risk in amplifying real economy shocks. Household credit is highly vulnerable to major declines in household income. Unemployment is a major factor in declines in household income, although this can be buffered by government income transfer policies. Sudden increases in regional unemployment lead to credit stresses, especially in consumer credit and mortgages. This in turn leads to increases in loan losses for financial institutions and, in extreme cases, failures of financial institutions. The GFC was an excellent example of the consequences of mortgage losses for unemployment, consumer spending, and wealth.[37]

During this pandemic, government subsidies have reduced credit losses. In addition, post-GFC reforms and regulations on bank balance sheets have implied limited stress for banks and credit markets. Financial regulators have been monitoring the banking sector during the pandemic watching for weaknesses in the system that could be avoided by new regulatory action.[38]

Corporate leverage and revenue declines lead to increased risks of corporate defaults. As firms see major declines in working capital, banks must attempt the difficult task of calculating loan losses contingent on government lockdown and recovery policies. These risks are compounded by the uncertainty surrounding various government loan subsidy programs, as well as pressure from bank regulators to relax prudent lending practices. As government policies in this area have changed rapidly, with considerable ambiguity, bank compliance departments and boards faced unenviable decisions.

Government loan policies are problematic as they increase corporate and household leverage and default risk, unless some of the government-subsidized debt will be forgiven or interest rates are below (preexisting) market rates, i.e., it is an effective subsidy. Any subsidy should be ex-ante explicit so that private agents are not exposed to credit risks arising from uncertainty over the duration and size of subsidies that are difficult to compute with any accuracy.

5.7 *The limitations of conventional macroeconomic and monetary modeling*

Conventional macroeconomic modeling uses negative "shocks" to drive declines in aggregate economic activity. The GFC demonstrated that these

---

[37] For example, see Mian and Sufi (2014) for a summary of the empirical evidence.
[38] For example, see the recent discussion and reports at the BIS, https://www.bis.org/speeches/sp210420.pdf; https://www.fsb.org/wp-content/uploads/P010421-1.pdf.

models were too aggregated and limited to deal with some of the most damaging effects of major credit losses to an economy. Microeconomic and financial details are critical in formulating policy responses to such external events.[39]

To illustrate this argument, consider the following example. A major disruption to the real economy may *not* create a major banking crisis. That depends on the degree of leverage in the financial system, and on the efficiency of the bankruptcy system. Consider an economy that has very low consumer, corporate, and bank leverage, i.e., high equity capital ratios. Then, consider a major decline in income for the real economy. Firms and households will suffer large equity losses long before defaults flow onto bank balance sheets.

Conversely, assume high financial leverage. Then, moderate declines in income will create credit stresses in the financial system, appearing directly on bank balance sheets. If the bankruptcy resolution systems work quickly and efficiently for public companies, this will reduce economic losses that would have been induced by lengthy and uncertain resolution procedures. For private companies and individuals who are largely reliant on bank loans, the effectiveness of banks in speedy resolutions will minimize additional economic losses and reduce the impact of the initial shock.[40] Corporate bankruptcy systems, if they are inefficient in dealing with resolutions, can introduce another layer of real losses, destroying economic value. Small businesses and consumers who become bankrupt can create value losses if banks and other creditors create inefficiencies in the resolution process.[41]

The losses imposed on the real economy are redistributed through the financial system to equity and debt claimants. At the same time, government policies will attempt to redistribute the real losses via subsidies, taxes, and government borrowing to reduce inequality. The ultimate incidence of the losses will be transferred across classes of agents now and in the future in ways that can be difficult to compute with any accuracy — especially in a crisis.

---

[39] For example, see Kay and King (2020, Chapters 19 and 20). They discuss the limitations of standard Macro-Money models and their poor track record in many crises.

[40] These additional losses are sometimes described as "amplifiers."

[41] See Crean and Milne (2022) forthcoming for a detailed discussion.

As we discussed in Chapter 4 in Section 4, another industry that is vulnerable to major economic disruptions is the insurance industry. For example, a major earthquake on the West Coast of North America would create major property insurance claims.[42] But, what may surprise many analysts are the major insurance claims for business disruption and cancellation or postponement of major events. Contracts have had definitional problems, creating confusion and legal claims by businesses. Lloyds of London estimated 2020 underwriting losses, as a result of COVID-19, to be approximately USD107 bn.[43]

The insurance industry and related government policy play an important role in dealing with catastrophic risks. In a world with full insurance markets, with government backstops for extreme events, the losses would be borne much more equally across the populace, due to diversification. But, if insurance markets are incomplete or function poorly, economic losses can be concentrated on a segment of the population with severe consequences for their economic welfare. In turn, these losses can impact the banking system and other related sectors.[44]

Since the GFC, economists have been constructing models that are more disaggregated. These models should be tested against the experience of the pandemic and its associated policies that have led to major economic contractions. How did the models correspond to the evidence observed during the pandemic? Were they useful in informing policy actions?

5.8 *Thinking through the microeconomics of pandemic disruptions*

A pandemic will heavily impact the health care and economic system. The appropriate actions require careful ex-ante planning to prepare the critical linkages which will come under stress. Highly restrictive lockdown policies that are enforced for several months will impact different sectors of

---

[42] See Le Pan (2016) and Crean and Milne (2022).

[43] See BBC May 2020, https://www.bbc.co.uk/news/business-52659313?intlink_from_url=&link_location=live-reporting-story.

[44] See Crean and Milne (2022) for a detailed discussion.

an economy with varying intensity, often in subtle ways that are not obvious for policymakers relying on conventional highly aggregated macroeconomic models. Here are some disparate examples observed over the first few months of the pandemic:

(a) 90% of Western medications are manufactured in China. Careful analysis should have revealed ex-ante scenarios where this supply chain would create major strategic stresses in the medical system.

(b) Lockdown policies can induce severe economic supply chain disruptions for manufacturing, commerce, and consumers. This is true regionally, nationally, and internationally.

(c) Australia typically had three weeks reserve of gasoline and aviation fuel. A disruption of international fuel supply chains would have severe economic and social consequences. For many years, senior Australian officials have complained about this strategic risk, but they were ignored by the politicians. The current government rushed to respond in the early months of the pandemic.[45] The COVID-19 crisis has drawn attention to underlying risks that had been previously ignored.

(d) Universities that rely heavily on Full-Fee-Paying international students suffered large losses and disruption from international quarantine regulations. Many of those universities had not considered these consequences in their planning.[46]

(e) Some countries (e.g., Australia and New Zealand) or regions with typically high immigration rates prior to the pandemic, that supported rapidly expanding and high-priced real estate markets, suffered falls in house prices and residential construction. Coupled with increased unemployment, credit losses can rise quickly, adversely impacting consumer, business, pension funds, banking, and shadow bank balance sheets.

(f) In the US, Australia, and New Zealand, there was a major shift in real estate demand away from some inner cities toward suburbs and

---

[45] https://www.aspistrategist.org.au/in-a-crisis-australians-might-soon-be-running-on-empty-2/.

[46] See Beach and Milne (2019).

smaller cities and towns. This led to large real estate price falls for inner cities and large price increases in suburbs and towns. The latter locations are favored by professionals who are able to work remotely.[47] Whether this structural change will be sustained is an open question.

6. The Case for Wargame Preparation for Future Pandemics

Many governments have struggled with the implications of the Coronavirus pandemic. Clearly, most Western countries were poorly prepared and scrambled to respond. Taiwan, Singapore, Japan, and South Korea have historical experience with viruses emanating from China. They evolved far less disruptive policies and responses during 2020. Their policy responses have not been perfect, but their preparation and experience during the current crisis should be studied very carefully.

A common element in policy strategies for these countries has been a rapid imposition of quarantine and/or banning international travel from infected areas; social distancing and the use of masks; and a widespread use of testing and contact tracing. They avoided strong lockdown policies.[48]

While these strategies worked in 2020 and for the first half of 2021, the emergence of the far more contagious Delta variant of the COVID Virus created significant problems for Japan with surging infection rates in August 2021.[49] The reasons for this surge are not clear at the time of writing.

---

[47] There have been numerous discussions in Australia and New Zealand about credit losses relating to real estate price declines in the inner city apartment market due to the collapse of immigration and population moving to outer suburbs and smaller cities. The New Zealand and Australian Federal governments effectively closed their national borders. Some Australian states closed their states borders for months.

[48] For a detailed discussion, see https://globalhealth.duke.edu/news/how-some-asian-countries-beat-back-covid-19.

[49] See https://www.japantimes.co.jp/news/2021/08/27/national/coronavirus-tracker-august-27/.

Australia and New Zealand followed a similar strategy, but imposed very restrictive rules on international travel into and out of their countries. In addition, many of the Australian states imposed a series of strict lockdowns that have created severe economic and social costs. An unfortunate consequence of the "fortress" mentality was a complacency and tardiness in rolling out vaccinations. By August 2021, the Delta variant of the virus gained a foothold in both countries and they faced surging cases.[50] In Australia, the resulting strong lockdowns for a majority of the population had predictable impacts on the economy.[51]

Health care authorities should have tested procedures for dealing with pandemic surges. These procedures should be stress tested and wargamed regularly to incorporate the latest techniques and strategies. Table-top exercises are good first steps, but more detailed stress tests and periodic full wargames are necessary for adequate preparation.

Although pandemics have been wargamed by health care authorities in the past, as far as can be determined from public documents, there was no adequate gaming of economic, financial, and fiscal consequences depending upon policy responses. The economic, social, strategic, fiscal, and political implications of quarantine policies can have very adverse long-run effects on private wealth, unemployment, and government balance sheets. Some effects are obvious; but just as important are the subtle effects that flow through the economic structure of the economy. In turn, economic disruption would flow through into financial markets, and through banking systems into credit losses. Inherent economic/financial weaknesses will act as amplifiers to the initial impact of quarantine policies.

Governments have acted to reduce private sector losses by providing very large fiscal and financial assistance to the private sector. But, it is apparent that at times these responses have been not planned properly, with significant inconsistencies and waste. Careful wargame preparation should have reduced these inefficiencies.

---

[50] See https://www.spectator.co.uk/article/prison-island-australias-covid-fortress-has-become-a-jail.

[51] https://www.wsj.com/articles/australia-already-in-recession-as-economic-slump-deepens-cba-says-11630049270.

6.1 *Preparing a health and economic pandemic stress test*

Because there have been exercises prior to the current COVID pandemic, a stress test should build upon that experience. The test would construct a pandemic scenario incorporating recent lessons. As we have explained in Chapter 4 (Section 5.3), an evaluation agency would check the availability of supplies, availability of important information at the local, national, and international governmental levels, etc. But, in addition, mimicking the lessons from the GFC, there should be pandemic stress tests that explore health, economic, financial, and budgetary consequences of a major pandemic and possible policy responses. The stress testing group could fall under the governance structure of the pandemic planning agency described in Chapter 4, but would need to include some independent outside experts. It should draw on experts drawn from health, economic, financial, and government budgetary agencies. Given that the stress tests would be run regularly, it is important that its composition is a rolling cadre of members who will draw on the experience of previous tests.

For pandemic preparations, the stress test group should draw on the most recent information and past experience to create a scenario fundamentally different from what has happened in the recent past. This could include an assumed new disease, spread in a particular way, affecting certain age groups, with a particular degree of transmissibility, the effectiveness of recent vaccine technology and its flexibility in adapting to a new virus and subsequent mutations, vaccine production capacity, and lags in production. It is critical that the stress test should include the social, economic, budgetary, and additional health consequences of government policies (e.g., the full consequences of regional and/or national lockdowns over a specific period of time.) One or two outside-the-box thinkers should be involved in the team putting together the stress test scenario.

The entire stress test should be revealed at once and officials should be given sufficient time to work through all the implications in some detail. Weaknesses of current plans should be noted and recommendations to improve them should be made.

Follow-up of those recommendations is essential. As we made clear in Chapter 4, an effective governance structure is critical in ensuring the lessons from stress test are incorporated into pandemic planning, procedures, and operations.

As we have emphasized above, the stress test should incorporate the preparation and effectiveness of different policies on social, economic, financial, and fiscal sectors of society. In particular, the stress test should incorporate testing the health, social, and economic consequences of various quarantine strategies, the availability of vaccines, and various medical treatments that can ameliorate serious medical conditions.

For example, in Canada, a pandemic stress test group would require the participation of senior officials from the Public Health Agency of Canada, the departments of health and finance, as well as the Bank of Canada and the bank regulator.

An important variation on the standard stress test would be to introduce a *cascading* stress test where the scenario began at the international level and then worked down to the national, regional, and local levels. This type of stress test would be most instructive for pandemics which spread widely across borders. These major international stress tests could be run every four or five years, mimicking the FSAP stress tests run by the IMF.[52]

One possibility for running this test would be for an international body to construct a pandemic scenario. This would be delivered to national health bodies who, with significant input from economic, financial, and social authorities, would use the scenario to test preparedness at the national, state/provincial, and local levels. One significant component of the test would require international cooperation on border quarantine, cross-border travel restrictions, and related strategies. Since the GFC, there have been significant advances in creating and strengthening international bodies to deal with financial stability: The pandemic stress test could use those resources as one part of the international pandemic stress test. The Financial Stability Board could supervise financial stability issues that would arise during the stress test scenario; the Committee on the Global Financial System at the Bank for International Settlements could explore monetary policy issues; the OECD could explore fiscal

---

[52] These international tests would not preclude more frequent national, provincial, and local stress tests.

issues arising in advanced countries; and the IMF could look at those same issues in other countries.

The cascading stress test would mimic a pandemic as it flowed across jurisdictions, testing cooperation, preparedness, and information systems at the global, national, and local levels. Scenario construction and stress test organization would require international cooperation similar to the international structures developed for the economic and financial system after the GFC.

Pandemic stress tests suffer the same limitations as financial stress tests: They omit the element of personal interaction over time as decision-makers and the public adjust their behavior to new information and situations that can be described as unintended consequences. Pandemic and policy responses create complex interactions across the health, social, economic, and fiscal areas of the economy. One approach to address this complexity is to run periodic wargames that require decision-makers to confront the dynamics of a complex societal problem. The dynamic aspect of these exercise might be described as "iterated stress tests" where the one-shot stress test is repeated over a number of iterations, taking the conclusion of the previous stress test as the starting point for a new test.

6.2 *Preparing a health and economic pandemic wargame*

In planning a pandemic wargame, one should draw on the long experience of wargaming methodology and knowledge that we outlined earlier in this chapter.

The wargame should use the experience of past health stress tests and wargames, improving their methodology, drawing on the lessons that we have learned in the COVID-19 episode. As we observed earlier, the earlier wargames did not provide adequate preparation for a pandemic. A major review should aim to improve health wargames and the health preparations for periodic pandemics.

Periodic wargames would test the institutional structures, procedures, and the effectiveness of key decision-makers. Regular wargames train existing and new decision-makers in the latest procedures. A system-wide wargame allows decision-makers in different organizations to become familiar with the key players, so that in a real pandemic, communication channels that have been forged in the wargame reduce confusion and increase the efficiency of decision-making and implementation.

The administrative structure that we outlined for an international or national cascading stress test could be used for constructing wargames. As the various administrative levels become used to wargame methodology and procedures, they can be used for focused training for key senior decision-makers. The relative frequency of stress tests versus wargames will depend upon their effectiveness, availability of key personnel, and resources and budgets.

Such a wargame will be a costly exercise if it is done properly. But, the costs of poor preparation are now only too evident. Regular wargames can reduce the costs of a real pandemic.

In the next subsections, we discuss some issues that have become apparent during this pandemic and should be incorporated into the combined game.

6.3 *Government communication policies are of critical importance*

Communication policies are critical in managing public information and combatting rumors, lies, and panic. These effects should be incorporated into systemic wargames. Social media and conventional media can amplify rumors and spurious stories, generating public panic and political pressure, inducing poor political policy choices. This does not imply that genuine open debate should be stifled — an open, informed analysis is crucial in formulating good policy. Government communication should be timely and avoid ambiguity. Where there is underlying uncertainty, governments should convey that information and explain the consequences for policies. The following example illustrates this argument.

6.3.1 *An example of uncertainty associated with an effective vaccine*

A good example of uncertainty is the discovery and introduction of a vaccine for the COVID-19 virus. The timing of an effective vaccine is fraught with uncertainty. Consider three scenarios that could be incorporated into a wargame. The first scenario describes a situation where an effective vaccine will be fully operational within a very short time span (e.g., three months). Now, this scenario will provide incentives to have a short, strong lockdown policy to flatten the curve, because the economic and social costs will be relatively small. Conversely, assume that a vaccine will take years to become operational. Now, this situation could provide incentives for a sequence of strong lockdown policies with intervening relaxations, or conversely, a more restrained lockdown or quarantine policy that is less socially and economically costly, hoping that herd immunity and more benign virus mutations will eventually reduce the spread and the lethality of the virus.

A more realistic scenario considers the two previous scenarios with the subjective likelihoods associated with each scenario. Policymakers face a difficult situation, where a strategy taken with all due care ex ante can appear to be incompetent with hindsight.

Given the development of mRNA vaccines for the virus, there is a strong possibility that future mutations or the emergence of other viruses can be combatted by rapidly developing appropriate mRNA vaccines within a short period of time. This possibility should be introduced as a serious contingent strategy that should be very effective for combatting the new virus and greatly reducing social disruption and economic costs.

6.4 *Developing communication policies for contingent strategies*

The previous example makes clear the uncertainty facing policymakers. What does this imply for communication strategies? Ambiguity and uncertainties should be communicated to the public as clearly as possible. Policies contingent on current and evolving information should be explained carefully to avoid the impression of incompetence that is tempting with 20–20 hindsight.

Given that, early in the COVID-19 crisis, there was great uncertainty regarding the degree and severity of the virus, the impact on various demographics, and the effectiveness of various treatments, policy communication should have outlined simple contingent policy responses. Although many governments attempted such contingent communication strategies, there were many examples of vacillation and changing objectives (mission creep in military jargon). A good example of the latter was the evolution in some jurisdictions of a policy of "flattening the infection curve" into "eradication of the virus."[53] Why this policy objective evolved was never made clear.

Errors should be acknowledged in a timely fashion. Correction of errors and updating strategies as new information becomes available should be explained carefully so that the public is informed. It is critical that contingent strategies be explained carefully and reinforced in the media. Sensible queries and questions from the media and public should not be brushed aside but answered honestly.

There are too many examples in various countries where strategies have been changed without adequate explanation, leading to public confusion and loss of trust in the authorities. Political and bureaucratic dissembling and confusion will erode trust. Once public trust is lost, the public will be open to manipulation by unscrupulous political operators and demagogues who exploit confusion to further their political agendas.

Economic rent seekers will attempt to shape policy to their advantage. With great uncertainty over possible treatments, the effectiveness of specialized equipment, exemptions from lockdowns, etc., rent seekers have incentives to exploit the media, pushing politicians into making imprudent expenditures and policies. The rent seekers should be exposed to the public.

Unscrupulous journalists and political opportunists will use sensationalism and the usual battery of dishonest tricks to attract fame and political leverage. All sorts of bizarre claims and policies have been advocated by fringe political activists and websites. They attempt to gain

---

[53] The latter objective is effectively impossible in the near term. Governments that boasted that they had eradicated the virus faced subsequence outbreaks — and embarrassing questions of competence. The State of Victoria in Australia is a classic example. The State government boasted that they had fully contained the virus with tough lockdown policies. Subsequently, international traveller quarantine procedures were bungled, creating a dangerous surge in virus infections and a dramatic reintroduction of a strong lockdown. The State government faced accusations of incompetence.

traction by fostering panic. This behavior is hardly new. The best remedy is exposure by a calm government which refuses to be panicked.

During a pandemic, hostile countries will attempt to use social media to sow distrust and panic to weaken a government and the country's economy and strategic position. They too should be exposed using credible information and the public warned of their nefarious activities. In certain extreme cases, such websites could be banned on the domestic web or at least signaled to the reader in a bold statement as the site appears.[54]

6.5 *The results of a pandemic wargame: What happens to the results?*

Having carefully constructed and executed a wargame, the results should be analyzed, reported, and acted upon to correct equipment and employee deficiencies, change organizational structures, and improve plans and procedures at international, national, state/provincial, and local levels. Lessons learned must be fed back up the system so that insights and successes at lower levels are recognized and circulated across the system so that successful innovations can be implemented by other authorities in the system. A similar response should be enacted to observations of failures, so that revised policies can be implemented.

Wargames should be played regularly to test new systems and technologies for their resilience under stress. New risks and uncertainties appear periodically — they should be wargamed in an attempt to locate weaknesses or inconsistencies with existing procedures. For example, the rapid development and deployment of mRNA vaccines have had a major impact on COVID-19 policies in reducing restrictions that had heavy social and economic costs. For similar viral epidemics, wargames should incorporate rapid vaccine development and deployment. For the economic wargame component, one could test the development of more effective, targeted insurance schemes, thus reducing future large fiscal burdens.

Complacency is dangerous. Major unexamined risks can be very costly as they impact unprepared systems and economies, inducing

---

[54] The most sophisticated operations by foreign adversaries will attempt to hide the real source of their attack. There are ways of combatting these types of operations.

panicked and very costly responses. Areas of weakness will require strengthening and periodic testing for compliance. It is incompetent to let careful reports gather dust, ignoring the lessons that have been observed in previous crises or exercises. A one-size-fits-all approach is not appropriate: Each weakness will require an appropriate remedy.

It is critical that the results of stress tests and wargames be summarized by a group *independent* of the participants in the exercise and likely including a number of those who created the stress test or wargame. They — or a related group — should review actions — importantly including changes in the official pandemic plans — taken from recommendations in the game summary. That review should take place within a year while the analysis is still fresh in the minds of the participants. Lack of action should be reported publicly together with the revised pandemic plan and an explanation why any recommendations were not adopted. The greatest danger is that bureaucratic lethargy, turnover of experienced players, etc., can blunt the lessons and dilute future preparation. As time passes, history is forgotten and the crises are neglected — until another crisis arises with its panicked, costly response.

6.6 *Training for pandemic, economic, and financial wargames*

Currently, many policy economists are woefully unprepared for this type of analysis. Few understand sophisticated strategic wargaming methods that have been developed and used by foreign policy, strategic, and military analysts. Also, most macroeconomists or monetary economists in government policy organizations do not understand the complexity and limitations of financial risk management practices used by the financial sector and regulators.

Similarly, the health policy establishment has only a rudimentary training in appropriate economic and financial theory and practice. Risk management is seen, far too often, as being highly specialized for banking and financial institutions and their regulators — and not relevant for many other social and economic policy areas.

These weaknesses should be addressed by requiring appropriate courses and training. This training should be regarded as a serious prerequisite for bureaucratic and political policymakers.

The COVID-19 pandemic has provided graphic examples of uncoordinated risk management and planning failures across medical, social, economic, financial, and government fiscal sectors. Far too often, policies appear to have been developed in specialist medical/pandemic policy silos, with scant understanding or interest of the social, economic, and financial consequences. When the social, economic, and financial costs became apparent, governments responded with subsidy schemes of various types. As we have observed above, the limitations of some of these hurried schemes have been revealed.

Coordinated wargaming for health, social, and economic systems would have made these limitations more apparent prior to a crisis, requiring careful preparation of playbooks and systems. Regular wargames should involve not only public and private sector professionals[55] but also government decision-makers, so that they understand the costs and benefits of policies, and the strengths and weaknesses of their procedures. They need to understand the crucial role of managing uncertainty and the importance of public communication to avoid panic and nefarious activities which exploit weakness and fear.

7. Conclusion

There has been a clear lack of preparation by many countries in dealing with the COVID-19 virus epidemic. The resultant economic and social costs have been very large. Policy decisions were taken under considerable uncertainty about the virulence and lethality of the virus. The consequences of this uncertainty could have been reduced by playing wargames so that policymakers were better prepared.

---

[55] Both private and public professionals should be carefully screened to avoid conflict-of-interest issues. They should be chosen for their expertise and ability for independent analysis of complex issues.

Although pandemic wargames had been played in the past, and reports on previous pandemics written, in most cases there appears to have been little action taken to implement lessons learned, or the creation of effective and cost-efficient responses. We have argued that preparation for pandemic and other major exogenous events will require regular wargames. Previous exercises have been too limited and have not considered very important social, economic, financial, and fiscal factors that have become apparent in the current crisis. These games or exercises should include medical, social, political, economic, and financial components that prepare various agents in these sectors for a major systemic event. Coordination and cooperation in these sectors are critical in managing a crisis.

The results from wargames should be summarized by an *independent* group within a year while the analysis is still fresh in the minds of the participants. The results should be available publicly for critical examination by experts in associated fields.

One important role of wargames is to train individuals and organizations to prepare them for emergencies. This educative process must be conducted regularly to avoid loss of corporate and organizational memory. Authorities should explore appropriate public communication strategies to reduce confusion and panic.

References

Adam, D. (2020). "Special Report: The Simulations Driving the World's Response to COVID-19: How Epidemiologists Rushed to Model the Coronavirus Pandemic," *Nature*, April 3, 2020, pp. 316–318.

Allen, T. (1987). *War Games: The Secret World of the Creators, Players, and Policy Makers Rehearsing World War III Today*. McGraw-Hill, New York.

Allen, T. (2015). *Thomas Allen's War Games Professional Wargaming 1945–1985*. Lulu Publishing, North Carolina.

Beach, C. and Milne, F. (2019). "Ontario Post-Secondary Education Funding Policies: Perverse Incentives and Unintended Consequences," QED Working Paper No. 1424. https://www.econ.queensu.ca/sites/econ.queensu.ca/files/wpaper/qed_wp_1424.pdf.

BIS Report (2017). "Supervisory and Bank Stress Testing: Range of Practices." https://www.bis.org/bcbs/publ/d427.pdf.

Buckner, D. and Dowd, K. (2021). "How Strong are British Banks? And Can They Pass the COVID-19 Stress Test?" Institute of Economic Affairs, Briefing, July 10, 2021.

Burrows, O., Learmonth, L. and McKeown, J. (2012). "RAMSI: A Top-down Stress-testing Model Developed at the Bank of England," *Bank of England Quarterly Bulletin*, Q3.

Carney, M. (2021). *Value(s): Building a Better World for All*. Signal Books, New York.

Crean, J. and Milne, F. (2022). "Covid and Other Catastrophes: Systemic Risks Neglected by Financial System Reform," Working Paper forthcoming.

Crouhy, M., Mark, R. and Galai, D. (2000). *Risk Management*. McGraw-Hill, New York.

Curry, J. and Drage, N. (2020). *The Handbook of Cyber Wargames*. The History of Wargaming Project. www.wargaming.co.

Dent, K., Westwood, B. and Segoviano, M. (2016). "Stress Testing of Banks: An Introduction," *Bank of England Quarterly Report*, Q3.

Dowd, K. (2005). *Measuring Market Risk*. (2nd Ed.), Wiley, New Jersey.

Dowd, K. (2014). "Math Gone Mad: Regulatory Risk Modelling by the Federal Reserve." Cato Institute.

Dowd, K. (2016). "No Stress: The Flaws in the Bank of England's Stress Testing Programme." Adam Smith Institute.

Ellison, G. (2020). "Implications of Heterogeneous SIR Models for Analyses of COVID-19," NBER Working Paper No. 27373, June.

Fique, J. (2017). "The MacroFinancial Risk Assessment Framework (MFRAF), Version 2.0," Bank of Canada. https://www.bankofcanada.ca/wp-content/uploads/2017/09/tr111.pdf.

Green, T. (2021). *The Covid Consensus: The New Politics of Global Inequality*. Hurst and Company, London.

Hershkovitz, S. (2019). "Wargame Business: Wargames in Military and Corporate Settings," *Naval War College Review*, 72(2), Spring 2019.

Horn, J. (2011). "Playing War Games to Win," *McKinsey Quarterly*, March 1, 2011. https://www.mckinsey.com/business-functions/strategy-and-corporate-finance/our-insights/playing-war-games-to-win.

Ioannidis, J. (2020). "Coronavirus Disease 2019: The Harms of Exaggerated Information and Non-Evidence-Based Measures," Editorial, *European Journal of Clinical Investigation,* 50(4), April, 5 pages.

Ioannidis, J., Cripps, S. and Tanner, M. (2020). "Forecasting for Covid-19 has Failed," International Institute of Forecasters, June. https://forecasters.org/blog/2020/06/14/forecasting-for-covid-19-has-failed/.

Kay, J. and King, M. (2020). *Radical Uncertainty: Decision-Making Beyond the Numbers*. Norton, New York.

Kirchoff, C. (2016). https://assets.documentcloud.org/documents/6817684/NSC-Ebola-Lessons-Learend-Report-FINAL-8-28-16.pdf.

Kirchoff, C. (2020). https://www.statnews.com/2020/03/24/chris-kirchhoff-ebola-coronavirus-response/.

Kubarych, R. (2001). *Stress Testing the System: Simulating the Global Consequences of the Next Financial Crisis*. Council on Foreign Relations Press, New York.

Le Pan, N. (2016). "Fault Lines: Earthquakes, Insurance, and Systemic Financial Risk." C. D. Howe Commentary No. 454. https://www.cdhowe.org/sites/default/files/attachments/research_papers/mixed/Commentary%20454_0.pdf.

Mian, A. and Sufi, A. (2014). *House of Debt: How They (and You) Caused the Great Recession, and How We Can Prevent It from Happening Again*. University of Chicago Press, Chicago.

Milne, F. (2008). "Anatomy of the Credit Crisis: The Role of Faulty Risk Management Systems," C.D. Howe Institute Commentary, No. 269. https://www.cdhowe.org/sites/default/files/attachments/research_papers/mixed//commentary_269.pdf.

Milne, F. (2009). "The Complexities of Financial Risk Management and Systemic Risks," *Bank of Canada Review*, Summer. https://www.bankofcanada.ca/wp-content/uploads/2010/06/milne1.pdf.

Roussel, Y. *et al.* (2020). "SARS-CoV-2: Fear versus Data," *International Journal of Antimicrobial Agents*, 55(5), May 2020, 3 pages.

Royal Society of Canada (2020). Restoring Trust: COVID-19 and the Future of Long-Term Care. https://rsc-src.ca/en/restoring-trust-covid-19-and-future-long-term-care.

SARS Commission Report, Ontario (2008). http://www.archives.gov.on.ca/en/e_records/sars/report/v1.html.

Chapter 6

Conclusion

The COVID-19 pandemic revealed serious deficiencies in government and public health preparation around the world. Some governments were better prepared than others, but most responses were poorly thought through or poorly implemented, leading to increased death rates for the most vulnerable and avoidable increases in social and economic costs. Although previous pandemics had produced major reports and plans preparing for future pandemics, in many cases, governments ignored the recommendations and found themselves scrambling to respond to the COVID-19 pandemic. Careful analysis reveals that these previous reports and plans were limited to health issues and ignored any consequences of broader government responses — such as lockdowns, loans to businesses, and various types of transfers to individuals and businesses.

One might argue that this lack of pandemic preparation was an unfortunate extreme case that was not consistent with other well-managed extreme event preparation and execution. But, we argue that there are disturbing similarities with another example of bungled preparations for a major event. We outline the inadequate understanding, preparation, and early policy responses to the Global Financial Crisis (GFC) of 2007–2009. Numerous reports and analyses have revealed that financial regulators, central banks, and ministries of finance were ill prepared for the financial and economic consequences of the housing crashes in the United States and elsewhere. Since the GFC there have been major regulatory reforms to bank capital and liquidity ratios to make banks more resilient to large losses. In addition, regulators have run large-scale stress tests of the banking system looking for weaknesses in bank balance sheets. There are some methodological lessons to be learned from the GFC episode and the subsequent regulatory and policy actions.

We propose two major policy responses for the COVID-19 pandemic. The first is to require sophisticated postmortems that analyze the policy successes and failures from around the world, given that governments have tried a variety of responses to the pandemic and some have been far more extreme than others in various dimensions. (These postmortems have strong parallels in the reports and regulatory actions following the GFC by the Basel Committee on Banking Regulation, the Financial Stability Board, and other international financial regulatory bodies, as well as national governments and financial regulators.) These postmortems should not only explore health policies but also the battery of social and economic policies that were undertaken to complement the health policies. Importantly, the analysis should include pandemic planning and preparation failures and successes. The reports will be required to make recommendations for pandemic preparation guarding against future pandemics. Postmortems will also need to address major governance issues that ensure that the recommendations will be enforced and not ignored — as some reports have been in the past.

The second policy proposal is to introduce major pandemic stress tests and exercises (wargames). This proposal again parallels part of the post-GFC regulatory responses. Stress tests and the more demanding exercises/wargames will search for weaknesses in preparation and planning for pandemics. They should incorporate the latest research and innovations in epidemiology, pandemic planning, vaccine research and production, and economic, financial, and social consequences of policy actions. These exercises should be educative in training decision-makers to deal with low-probability but high-cost crises. These stress tests and exercises need to be carried out at all levels: international, national, state/provincial, local public health units, and even hospitals.

A major benefit of this approach is that it requires a system-wide analysis of a pandemic — or any other catastrophic risk (e.g., major earthquake, flood, or cyber attack). These exercises will begin with a pandemic and health response, but much of the subsequent economic and social content will have strong similarities to other types of catastrophes that require risk planning.

Index

no one institution looking at
overall financial stability, 55
pandemic wargame in 2019, 80
real estate market, pandemic
effects, 140–1
regulatory systems reform, 67–8
risky financial institution lending
practice and bankruptcy, 51,
53, 70
vaccination rate, 30
vaccine development and
ordering, 30
universities, 93, 140
unregulated or less-regulated entries,
effects of a crisis on, 58–9, 70–1
US forensic report on 2014–2015
Ebola pandemic, 79–80
US pandemic wargame in 2019, 80

vaccinations
delays in routine vaccinations of
children, 22
of disadvantaged groups, 28
of those residing in low-income
countries, 10, 31
vaccine development, 30, 91
diversification across potential
suppliers, 30
mRNA vaccine technology, 29,
89, 129–130, 147, 149
timing of effective vaccine
129–30, 146–7, 149
vaccine ordering, 29–30, 39
countries ill prepared for, 10
and domestic development,
Australia, 30
and international supply chain
problems, 52, 89
and "portfolio diversification",
Canada, 30, 54

vaccines
effectiveness, 94
G7 countries pledge supply of,
31
outsourcing of supplies, 52
uncertainties associated with an
effective vaccine, 146
wargame use over availability in
the pandemic, 129
Vancouver, major earthquake,
systemic wargame, 127
ventilators, 8–9, 12
Victoria
boasts about eradication of the
virus and subsequent out-
breaks, 148
breakdown in quarantine system,
52, 109–11
COVID policy and
implementation crisis, case
study, 109–11
COVID-19 hotel quarantine
inquiry, 110
deaths from COVID-19, 110
deaths in long-term care homes,
110
economic and social costs of
very restrictive lockdowns,
110
Vietnam, 19
"viral load" and transmission, 33, 36
viruses
contagious, and pandemics, 11
incentives to slow the spread,
130
and model development, 32–3
uncertainty about virulence and
lethality, 56, 112
virulent strains, 91
see also COVID-19 virus